D1357671

American Bioethics

George J. Annas

. . . .

AMERICAN
BIOETHICS

. . . .

Crossing Human Rights and
Health Law Boundaries

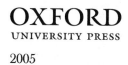

UNIVERSITY PRESS

2005

OXFORD
UNIVERSITY PRESS

Oxford   New York
Auckland   Bangkok   Buenos Aires   Cape Town   Chennai
Dar es Salaam   Delhi   Hong Kong   Istanbul   Karachi   Kolkata
Kuala Lumpur   Madrid   Melbourne   Mexico City   Mumbai   Nairobi
São Paulo   Shanghai   Taipei   Tokyo   Toronto

Copyright © 2005 by George J. Annas

Published by Oxford University Press, Inc.
198 Madison Avenue, New York, New York 10016

www.oup.com

Oxford is a registered trademark of Oxford University Press

Library of Congress Cataloging-in-Publication Data
Annas, George J.
American bioethics : crossing human rights and health law boundaries / George J. Annas.
p. cm.
Includes bibliographical references and index.
ISBN 0-19-516949-2
1. Human rights—Moral and ethical aspects.   2. Medical laws and legislation—Moral and
ethical aspects.   3. Medical laws and legislation—Moral and ethical aspects—United States.
4. Bioethics—United States.   I. Title.
K3240.A56 2004
174'.957'0973—dc22   2004045576

9 8 7 6 5 4 3 2 1

Printed in the United States of America
on acid-free paper

To Katie and David

and their generation of human rights and health advocates

Acknowledgments

American Bioethics continues my exploration of the relationships between bioethics and law begun in *Standard of Care: The Law of American Bioethics* and continued in *Some Choice: Law, Medicine, and the Market*. As with these earlier works, I benefited greatly from conversations, debates, comments, and criticisms of my colleagues in the Department of Health Law, Bioethics and Human Rights at the Boston University School of Public Health, most especially Leonard H. Glantz, Michael A. Grodin, Wendy K. Mariner, and Winnie Roche. We have been together for almost two decades, during which time we have together explored and crossed traditional academic boundaries, including those combined in our Department's new name and in this book. It has been terrific, and our Dean, Robert Meenan, has been a strong supporter of our work. I also greatly appreciate the consistent support of Jeffrey House of Oxford University Press for all three books.

Special thanks are due to Michael Grodin (again), with whom I founded Global Lawyers and Physicians, and with whom I have taught a course on "Human Rights and Health" for each of the past six years. Many of the ideas involving the new field of health and human rights grew out of this course, as well as our work with others in the field, especially the late Jonathan Mann, and our colleagues at the Harvard School of Public Health, Sofia Gruskin and Stephen Marks. An earlier version of Chapter 4 was coauthored with my colleagues Lori Andrews and Rosario Isasi, both of whom I continue to work with on issues of global governance of genetic technologies. I also get many ideas from my wife, Mary Annas, and our children, Katie and David, who give me some measure of confidence that their generation might not repeat many of the mistakes of mine. I am happy to dedicate this book to them. The exceptional staff of the Department of Health Law, Bioethics and Human Rights has always made manuscript preparation much smoother than it should be, and Emily Bajcsi was especially instrumental in the preparation of this book.

Earlier versions of most of the chapters in *American Bioethics*, Chapter 2 and Chapters 5 through 12, first appeared in the *New England Journal of Medicine*, and most of these were expertly edited by Marcia Angell. An earlier version of Chapter 3 appeared in the *Emory Law Review*, Chapter 4 in the *American Journal of Law & Medicine* (coauthored by Lori Andrews and Rosario Isasi), and Chapter 1 in Jonathan Moreno's *In the Wake of Terror*.

Contents

Concluding Remarks: Bioethics, Health Law,
    and Human Rights Boundary Crossings   159

"The voluntary consent of the human subject is absolutely essential."

—Nuremberg Code, 1947

"Everyone has the right to a standard of living adequate for the health and well-being of himself and his family, including food, clothing, housing and medical care and necessary social services. . . . Motherhood and childhood are entitled to special care and assistance."

—Universal Declaration of Human Rights, 1948

Introduction

"So you're a bio*ethna*cist," began Stephen Colbert as he opened his interview with medical historian David Rothman on Jon Stewart's *The Daily Show* in 2003, the 50th anniversary of the discovery of the structure of DNA. Rothman was being questioned, together with James Watson, about whether there is a "stupidity gene." Rothman insisted, "no, no, an *ethi*cist," to which Colbert responded curtly, "a bio . . . one of those things." Playing bioethics for laughs on *Comedy Central* is an indication both that bioethics has made it in America, and that it is in some danger of becoming a joke. On the serious side, President George W. Bush devoted his first major televised address to the nation to a bioethical issue (embryonic stem cell research) and his appointment of a President's Council on Bioethics with the broad charge to "consider all of the medical and ethical ramifications of biomedical innovation." On the more foolish side, Congress passed a bill (for the third time) criminalizing a medical procedure, so-called partial birth abortion, and the Florida legislature, with the endorsement of Governor Jeb Bush, passed a law requiring a feeding tube to be reinserted into a woman in a persistent vegetative state. American bioethicists have successfully promoted informed choice in the doctor–patient relationship, and were instrumental in promulgating federal regulations to protect research subjects; but ethics committees have had only limited success, and bioethicists have had little to say either about access to health care by tens of millions of uninsured Americans, or even about patient safety and medical malpractice.

These examples tell us a lot about American bioethics. First, bioethics has become a widely recognized field, complete with its own experts whose opinions matter. Presidents Carter, Reagan, Clinton, and Bush all felt it important to name their own "bioethicists" to national committees and commissions. Second, as these examples suggest, American bioethics is about much more than "ethics," it is about law and politics. That is why, more than a decade ago, I subtitled my *Standard of Care* "The Law of American Bioethics," noting that "American law, not philosophy or medicine, is primarily responsible for the agenda, development and current state of American bioethics." It was true then and remains true today. American bioethics is more pragmatic than principled. And to the extent that American bioethics has principles, they are mostly drawn from American law, including liberty (autonomy) and justice. Autonomy has a dark side, and in the context of America's market ideology can make choice seem like a legitimate end in itself regardless of the poverty of the available options, a theme I explored in *Some Choice: Law, Medicine, and the Market.* In this book I ask whether bioethics can regain its aspirational core and redeem itself from being just another legal or marketing specialty in America.

The perhaps surprising answer comes not from within bioethics, but from outside—and this time from beyond America itself, from the international human rights movement. There is certainly such a thing as international human rights law, but as set forth in the Universal Declaration of Human Rights, and even in two major subsequent treaties, it remains fair to characterize much of international human rights as aspirational in character. The most important development in bioethics in the past decade has been its movement toward globalization, and this will ultimately, I believe, require the fields of bioethics and human rights to work together. Luckily, the two fields have a natural symbiosis. The symbiosis of bioethics and human rights can be most clearly discerned in crimes against humanity that have historically involved physicians, such as torture, imprisonment, execution, and lethal human experimentation. More recently it can be seen, especially as exemplified by Médecins sans Frontières and Physicians for Human Rights, in physician movements to deliver essential medicines to all who need them and more broadly to make the "right to health" a reality globally.

What all this means is that even though Daniel Callahan is correct to describe bioethics as a "native grown American product," its future is likely to be increasingly international in character. Bioethics has always been concerned with power, especially the power physicians have historically had over patients and the power of new technologies to diagnose and treat disease. Mostly, beginning at Nuremberg and the Doctors' Trial, bioethics has been a reaction against the arbitrary use of power. Bioethics attempts, for example, to replace paternalism with informed choice and to make the right to refuse *any* medical intervention meaningful. Reactionary ethics, of course, comes too late, after the harm has been done. That is also the history of medicine, the treatment of disease and injury to alleviate pain and suffering in individuals. Public health, on the other hand, has had a different mission: the prevention of disease in populations. Just as medical ethics has developed to redistribute power in the doctor–patient relationship, so modern public health is struggling to articulate an ethics of its own. The struggle is ongoing, but a major contender for the ethics of human welfare that public health aspires to protect and promote is the Universal Declaration of Human Rights itself.

At the 50th anniversary of the deciphering of the structure of DNA, which also marks the completion of the sequencing of the human genome (the goal of the human genome project), the world is faced with a challenge and an opportunity. The code of the human genome is a scientific fact that should lead us to an understanding that all human beings are fundamentally the same. The opportunity is to use the knowledge of this scientific code together with the complementary values of the code of human rights, the Universal Declaration of Human Rights, for the betterment of all humans. To put it in somewhat reductionistic bioethics language, the genetic code is a fact-based code, and the human rights code is a value-based code. Facts cannot answer value questions, but they can inform them—and in this instance these two "universal" human codes reinforce and inform each other on the fundamental question of human equality and human rights.

The essays in this book explore specific questions in bioethics with a view toward crossing boundaries that have seemed to separate the field of bioethics from law, and more recently from human rights. These borders are permeable—and ultimately provide enclosures only to academics. In our increasingly globalized world, human rights will become the umbrella field under which the work done by both American bioethics and American health law will be linked and furthered.

The book is divided into two related parts. The first, "Bioethics and Human Rights," deals with some of the major human rights issues of our day and looks at them from a bioethics perspective, with heavy emphasis on American bioethics. It begins with 9/11 and the impact of terrorism on bioethics and moves to considerations of bioethics and human rights generally, the impact of new genetic technologies, international treaties and bioethics, the right to health, and finally the death penalty and moral progress. The second part, "Bioethics and Health Law," is focused on the bioethics and law boundary, but the attempt to confine a specific bioethics problem to a solution in American law is manifestly incomplete. The subjects considered are the ever fascinating quandary of separating conjoined twins when one will die, defining and enforcing patient rights, the role of law enforcement in the practice of medicine, the intractable (American) problem of abortion politics, the new reproductive technologies, and finally our fascination with illusions of immortality.

Of the 12 chapters that constitute this book, 9 have been adapted from articles that originally appeared in the *New England Journal of Medicine*, one from the *Emory Law Journal*, and one from the *American Journal of Law & Medicine*, and one, the first chapter, originally appeared as a chapter in a book written in response to 9/11. All have been updated to reflect the book's crossing boundaries theme. The concluding remarks were written for this book. The three primary human rights documents, as well as the Nuremberg Code, are included in the Appendixes.

Internationalism is out of fashion in America today, but isolation is not viable in a globalized world. Bioethics has tended to be more attuned to Huxley's *Brave New World,* with its vision of commodification and dehumanization of life, than to Orwell's *1984,* with its world based on perpetual war and fear. Our post-9/11 war on terrorism did not wipe out our concerns with dehumanization, as, for example, the President's Council on Bioethics 2003 report, *Beyond Therapy: Biotechnology and the Pursuit of Happiness*, underlines. Nonetheless, neat compartmentalization, within categories or within countries, is no longer an option. The world has become both more interdependent and more dangerous. We could wind up with a perverse combination of the worst features of both *1984* and *Brave New World,* or, by trying to avoid only one, wind up with the other.

American bioethics must expand its horizons, both geographically and contextually: boundaries must be crossed, and alliances formed. The next step for American bioethics is to become international and universal, not as an imperialist project, but as a learning project. The thesis of this book is that the framework and language of human rights, especially the Universal Declaration of Human Rights, provides American bioethics with a path to move forward. The challenge for American bioethicists is to work with international human rights advocates as partners in imaginative ways to help make the world a more just and healthier place for all of us to live.

Boston
July 4, 2004

I

. . . .

BIOETHICS AND HUMAN RIGHTS

1

. . . .

Bioethics and Bioterrorism

Amerian bioethics is often more pragmatic than principled, and quickly crossed both health law and human rights boundaries in response to 9/11 and our new global war on terrorism. War and terrorism test our commitment to principles, especially legal principles, and can cause us to temporarily abandon them. Although it has been three years since 9/11, health law, bioethics, and human rights lessons can already be drawn from America's reaction to this unprecedented terrorist atrocity.

Fear makes it difficult to distinguish fact from fiction, reality from fantasy, and truth from lies, all of which means that our initial reactions are likely to be overreactions that we will ultimately come to regret. In the immediate aftermath of 9/11 both bioethics and human rights principles were compromised in America. Nonetheless, the premise of this opening chapter is that boundary crossings between the realms of bioethics, health law, and human rights, tentatively under way well before 9/11, take on more urgency in its wake.[1] In fact, 9/11 itself could yet serve as a catalyst to bring these symbiotic fields even closer together—working synergistically to make the world a better place to live. Taking human rights, health law, and bioethics seriously makes the goals of health and safety of the public more realistic, at least in democracies where public trust in government is essential to success. 9/11 may be as important to the growth of American bioethics as World War II was to its birth.

Choosing Fantasy

It is a commonplace in science fiction that what cannot be understood is often seen as magic or miracle and arouses both fear and wonder. This is certainly true of much novel human experimentation. There is, nonetheless, a tendency to treat medical research and its claims as if they are all true, rather than to submit them to the skepticism of the scientific method, which requires proof, not just claims. At the other extreme, some people are willing to accept even the most sinister conspiracy theories and most bizarre accounts of present-day research. For example, in my last book, *Some Choice: Law, Medicine, and the Market,* I included an updated version of three of my dark, fictional pieces combined into Chapter 13. Titled "Our Most Important Product," in this reincarnation, it is an imagined transcript of a 1994 meeting of what I describe as a "top secret federal interagency group known as Perfect People 2020." The minutes include discussions not only of research projects to construct the perfect human (replacing the perfect soldier project) but also of implanting nonremovable monitoring and behavior modification devices in newborns, using comatose women as surrogate mothers for genetic experiments, providing additional funding to create humans with gills (projects to create people with wings and artificial wheels were temporarily suspended), as well as supporting an effort to capture 25 males and females from each of the world's "vanishing tribes" and relocate them to an island sanctuary for genetic variation research projects.[2]

     Even though the section on the human genome diversity project had earlier been rejected by *Nature* (the editor writing me that two of the four associate editors he had asked to read it thought it was a serious scientific proposal), I had not anticipated that readers would take Chapter 13 as fact (at least not for very long). Nonetheless, two reviewers of the book called me to ask about this chapter particularly, and another summarized the contents of every chapter except 13 in his review. And for the last five years I have regularly received e-mails from readers who are convinced that Chapter 13 is fact, not fiction. Some want to make sure I am still alive and in good health after divulging the existence of this secret group, but most want to know if I can help them get access to more minutes of the group or if I can tell them what it has been up to recently. Although I am fond of satire, it is almost impossible to write it in today's world, where almost anything you can think of is actually being proposed—or even attempted—by someone. With the revelation by the Bush administration that since 9/11 there has been a "shadow government" operating in secret bunkers outside Washington, I expect more e-mails, and I would not even be too surprised to learn that a Perfect People 2020–type committee actually exists. Nonetheless, let me assure readers that no attempt at satire appears in *American Bioethics*.

Two of the most popular movies immediately after 9/11 help illustrate our contemporary inability to distinguish (or want to distinguish) fantasy from reality: *Black Hawk Down* and *The Fellowship of the Ring*. Both movies were based on books, one about a factual event, the other pure fantasy, and they have similarities that help explain their post-9/11 popularity.

Black Hawk Down is the story of the 15-hour battle of Mogadishu, Somalia, in which American Rangers and Delta Force members fought off overwhelmingly larger Somali forces after two of their Black Hawk helicopters had been shot down. Eighteen American soldiers died in the battle. Two observations stand out for me, one from the finely reported book, the other from the more problematic movie. Mark Bowden, who interviewed most of the Americans involved in the battle, notes in the afterword to the paperback edition of his book:

> Their experience of battle, unlike that of any other generation of American soldiers, was colored by a lifetime of watching the vivid gore of Hollywood action movies. In my interviews with those who were in the thick of the battle, they remarked again and again how much they felt like they were *in a movie*, and had to remind themselves that this horror, the blood, the death, was real. They describe feeling weirdly out of place, as though *they did not belong here*, fighting feelings of disbelief, anger, and ill-defined betrayal. *This cannot be real*.[3]

This description will, of course, resonate with most Americans who watched the second plane hit the World Trade Center or who watched (and rewatched) the replays. Who didn't think, "This cannot be real"? The primary lesson of the movie was drawn by *Wall Street Journal* movie reviewer Joe Morgenstern, who reviewed the movie *We Were Soldiers* together with *Black Hawk Down*. He concluded that the message of both movies is best articulated by the narrator at the end of *Soldiers*: "In the end they fought not for their country or their flag, they fought for each other."[4]

The most popular and critically acclaimed movie immediately after 9/11 was based on J. R. R. Tolkien's *The Fellowship of the Ring*. The movie (which, like *Black Hawk Down*, closely follows the book) involves the quest by a fantasy character, the hobbit Frodo, who is chosen to attempt to destroy the ring of power before it can be used by an evil wizard to rule the world. Frodo, who is fearful of the task before him, laments in words that bring 9/11 to mind (and for this reason were used by the studio to promote the movie), "I wish it need not have happened in my time." Frodo's friend, the good wizard Gandalf, replies, "So do I and so do all who live to see such times. But that is not for them to decide. All we have to decide is what to do with the time that is given us."[5] There are many reasons for this movie's post-9/11 popularity, but the most likely explanation is that (like *Black Hawk Down*) it provides moviegoers with a good versus evil drama at a time when we really want to believe that we are the good guys fighting evil in the real world. Few were surprised when the final movie in the trilogy, *The Return of the King*, in which good triumphs over evil, dominated the 2004 Oscars with a record-tying eleven Academy Awards.

Good versus Evil

Terrorism is evil; human rights and bioethics are good. In a time of terror, when many Americans fear for their personal safety and that of their families, it seems reasonable to do what we can to protect ourselves and to permit (and even require) our government to do what seems necessary to protect us. One prominent bioethicist, for example, reacted to 9/11 by arguing that we are all soldiers now.[6] This implies the necessity for the type of solidarity exhibited by soldiers in the battles portrayed in *Black Hawk Down* and *We Were Soldiers*. A well-known health lawyer responded to 9/11 by proposing that states enact new bioterrorism quarantine laws that, among other things, would require American citizens to submit to examination and treatment by physicians or public health officials and require physicians and hospitals to do whatever public health officials tell them to do (including forced treatment) or face criminal prosecution or internment.[7] This is a classic good versus evil view of the world, but fantastically treats only public health officials as the good and Americans and their physicians (instead of the terrorists) as the evil enemy. In this fantasy, public health officials are to wear the ring of power themselves in times of emergency.

Is it true that we Americans must trade our human rights for safety to effectively fight terrorism? Must we, for example, dispense with the core value of modern bioethics, autonomy, in the face of a bioterrorist attack? I think the answer to both of these questions is no, and that trading rights for safety will leave us with neither. Far from having to compromise human rights and bioethical principles in time of terror, honoring these principles is likely to be our best defense against future terrorist attacks. Most specifically, taking the legal and ethical principle of informed consent seriously in the United States instills trust in government officials and makes the public much more likely to follow reasonable government advice in an emergency. Globally, promoting human rights, including the right to health, is likely to be the most effective action health care professionals can take to deter terror.

Three bioethics examples help illustrate how taking human rights seriously, even in times of national emergency, can be both the right policy and the most effective policy. They also illustrate the overlap, and thus potential merger, of bioethics and human rights, at least as they relate to health. Two of the examples are attempts to displace human rights for expediency, and the other illustrates an attempt (albeit a clumsy one) to respect human rights and bioethics. The examples are the Bush-Rumsfeld decision to ignore the Geneva Conventions for the al Qaeda and Taliban prisoners held at Guantanamo, the mini-Patriot Act proposal that states plan to force medical treatment on Americans in the event of a bioterrorist attack, and the government's offer of an investigational anthrax vaccine to those potentially exposed in the post-9/11 anthrax attacks.

Prisoners of War

The treatment of prisoners of war is the subject of the third of four Geneva Conventions, most recently revised in 1949, following World War II. The conventions are the core of international humanitarian law (the law of war) and also cover care of the wounded and sick as well as treatment of civilian populations. The United States has historically insisted that other countries follow the Conventions. Nonetheless, after transferring more than 100 al Qaeda and Taliban prisoners from Afghanistan to the U.S. Naval Base at Guantanamo, the United States took the position that the Geneva Conventions did not apply because the suspected terrorist "detainees" were not prisoners of war, but "unlawful combatants." On January 18, 2002, for example, President Bush decided both that the prisoners at Guantanamo would not be given POW status and that the United States would not abide by Geneva Convention III in their treatment.[8] Both decisions were wrong as a principled matter of human rights law and a pragmatic matter of effective policy.

The treatment of prisoners is, of course, a major human rights concern as well as a bioethics issue. Physicians have often been called on by prison officials to help maintain order by dispensing drugs and to help determine whether it is safe to continue torture or interrogation. All medical codes of ethics prohibit physicians from participating in torture in any way. And Article 13 of the Geneva Convention III states explicitly:

> Prisoners of war must at all times be humanely treated. . . . In particular, no prisoner of war may be subjected to physical mutilation or to medical or scientific experiments of any kind which are not justified by the medical, dental or hospital treatment of the prisoner concerned and carried out in his interest. Likewise, prisoners of war must at all times be protected, particularly against acts of violence or intimidation and against insults and public curiosity.[9]

In addition, Article 3, common to all four Conventions, prohibits "at any time and in any place . . . outrages upon personal dignity, in particular humiliating and degrading treatment." The United States was correct to argue that under the Geneva Conventions not everyone in military custody must be granted POW status, but the decision of who is and who is not a POW cannot be made arbitrarily. Instead, the Geneva Conventions require that all military prisoners have POW status until a "competent tribunal" determines that they are not in a category of persons protected by the convention (Article 5). Members of militias and organized resistance movements, for example, qualify for POW status if they are under command, have a distinctive sign recognizable at a distance, carry arms openly, and conduct their operations in accordance with the laws and customs of war (Article 4A). Because the United States brought the prisoners to Guantanamo for questioning, the provision of the convention that prohibits trying to force POWs to divulge more than their names, ranks, and serial numbers is probably the main one the United States sought to avoid.

The United States has endured a firestorm of international protests about the conditions of the prison camp at Guantanamo, the transportation of prisoners to it (at least one was drugged for the long plane trip, and all were shackled and blindfolded), and their initial housing in open cages.[10] It took a former military leader, Secretary of State Colin Powell, to try to impress upon President Bush how important the Geneva Conventions are to U.S. soldiers, who are, of course, subject to capture themselves and whom the U.S. military wants protected by the conventions.[11]

Americans themselves, however, did not seem to care very much how the prisoners were treated in the immediate aftermath of 9/11. David Letterman probably captured the mood of the country concerning the prisoners when he listed his top ten complaints by the prisoners at Camp X-ray (now Camp Delta): complaint number 10, "Three meals a day and none of them are goat," and number 4, "Achmed totally stole my skit idea for camp talent show." Bush partially relented. He decided that the Geneva Conventions did apply to the Guantanamo prisoners although he continued to insist that no prisoner would be given POW status. This latter decision, of course, is itself a violation of Article 5 of Geneva III and makes one wonder what the president understood by saying the conventions applied to the prisoners.[12]

In the end the United States is left looking like an unprincipled bully, a superpower that chose to ignore international law and human rights when it suited its purposes, even regarding treaties it has ratified. These actions severely undermine U.S. credibility in supporting human rights worldwide and unnecessarily put our own armed forces at much higher risk of not having the Geneva Conventions applied to them when captured by another country. During the three-week Iraq war in 2003, when American soldiers were captured, the president insisted that Iraqi military leaders would be held accountable if they did not follow the Geneva Conventions in caring for the prisoners of war. This "pick and choose" approach to human rights, of course, did not escape criticism. *Washington Post* cartoonist Tom Toles pictured Uncle Sam looking through the provisions of the Geneva Conventions and saying, "Here's one I like."

Taking human rights seriously in this context would have better sustained international support for the U.S. fight against terrorism. Moreover, following a convention-mandated screening process, the United States could lawfully have questioned those prisoners (likely a majority) who did not qualify for POW status under the conventions. In short, little was gained, and much was lost, in the administration's attempt to trash the Geneva Conventions by putting pragmatism over principle.

The administration's decision to treat the Geneva Conventions as inapplicable helped create a sense that Guantanamo was a legal black hole to which neither U.S. nor international law applied. This attitude in turn helped produce the scandalous abuse and torture of Iraqi prisoners of war at Abu Ghraib prison. The photographs of their humiliating and degrading treatment made it appear that the United States was willing to fight terror with terror. Abu Ghraib negated any American claim of moral superiority in the world and destroyed all human rights rationales for the Iraq war. The "good guys" had become the "evildoers" on prime-time TV for the world to see.

Military physicians performed better and honored both medical ethics and the human rights provisions of Geneva I, which covers wounded prisoners. After the fiercest battle in Afghanistan (part of Operation Anaconda), for example, the surgeon in command of the U.S. Army field hospital at Bagram Air Base, Lt. Col. Ronald Smith, told reporters who asked him that the Taliban and al Qaeda wounded were being treated side by side with the American wounded at the hospital, noting that "the ethics of combat surgery" require it.[13]

It is also worth noting that the Geneva Conventions themselves affirmatively protect medical ethics. For example, Article 16 of Protocol 1 (1977) states in relevant part:

1. Under no circumstances shall any person be punished for carrying out medical *activities compatible with medical ethics,* regardless of the person benefiting therefrom.
2. Persons engaged in medical activities shall not be compelled to perform acts or to cary out work contrary to the *rules of medical ethics* or to other medical rules designed for the benefit of the wounded and sick or to the provisions of the Conventions or this Protocol, or to refrain from performing acts or from carrying out work required by those rules and provisions. (emphasis added)

In short, under international humanitarian law, human rights and medical ethics requirements are symbiotic.

Preparing for Bioterrorism

About six weeks after 9/11, the Johns Hopkins-Georgetown Center for Law and the Public's Health announced that its lawyers had drafted a "model" state emergency bioterrorism law that, if enacted by the individual states, would permit the governor to put sweeping powers into the hands of public health officials in a public health emergency, such as a bioterrorist attack.[14] Among its provisions, all drawn from the existing laws of a variety of states in a "cut and paste" exercise, the act would make it a crime for members of the public to refuse to obey the orders of a public health official, including an order to be tested and an order to be vaccinated or treated. Physicians would also be subject to criminal penalties for not following the orders of a public health official to test or treat, and the orders of public health officials would be "immediately enforceable by any peace officer." Individuals who refused to be tested or treated could be immediately put in isolation or quarantine. Public health officials would be immune from civil action against them, even if they negligently caused death or serious personal injury.

These provisions, of course, are contrary to constitutional law, which, for example, gives individuals the right to refuse any treatment, as well as contrary to basic principles of medical ethics, which do not permit physicians to treat patients against their will or to treat patients in a manner the physician believes would be injurious to them, even under threat of criminal prosecution. What could have prompted lawyers at prominent academic institutions to react to 9/11 in a way that is blatantly anti-American (and anti-American bioethics) and, if anything, echoes the old Soviet system, in which public officials were given arbitrary and unaccountable power over citizens? The most likely answer is a combination of fantasy and fear. Both were combined in pre-9/11 role-playing "terrorism games" like TOPOFF (a hypothetical plague attack) and Dark Winter (a simulated hypothetical smallpox attack). The fear factor was multiplied on 9/11.

As Karl von Clausewitz noted in his treatise *On War*, at the outset of a war most information will be misinformation, "and the timidity of men gives fresh force to lies and untruths. As a general rule, everyone is more inclined to believe the bad than the good. Everyone is inclined to magnify the bad in some measure. . . ."[15] This certainly seems to be the case here, and the authors of the October 23, 2001, "model" bill very soon retreated from their initial proposal.

The cover page of the October 23 version stated that it was prepared "for" the Centers for Disease Control and Prevention (CDC) and "in collaboration with" many national organizations. In addition, chief drafter Lawrence Gostin told *USA Today* that his proposal was "strongly endorsed" by Department of Health and Human Services (DHHS) Secretary Tommy Thompson.[16] Gostin also told the *Johns Hopkins Public Health Magazine* that the act was "polished and strong because we had a brain trust of the best public health minds at Hopkins and the best legal minds at Georgetown, thus ensuring the best dividends for the nation."[17]

This was wishful thinking at best. Faced with public criticism, the authors retreated to revise their "polished product." A revised version of the "model" act was made available on December 21. Labeled "a draft for discussion" and prepared not "in collaboration with" but rather simply "to assist" the organizations previously listed, no one any longer, implicitly or explicitly, endorsed the "model" act, even the authors themselves. Most telling, the new cover page contained an explicit disclaimer.[18]

Even though representing no one's views and contrary to most law professors' views that it should not be taken seriously, the draft nonetheless took on a life of its own and has required considerable work on the part of members of the New England Coalition for Law and Public Health and other patient and consumer advocacy groups to explain why its draconian provisions are not only unnecessary but counterproductive.[19] The authors themselves have been helpful in this regard. Codrafter Steve

Teret, for example, explained that he had just finished reading José Saramago's *Blindness* when asked to help on this draft. He told an interviewer that the horrific quarantine described in this fictional epidemic of blindness was something he could not get out of his mind. In his words, "It was the most disturbing book I've ever read."[20] Of course, fiction often is more informative than nonfiction, especially in leading us to think about the future. Nonetheless, the drafters ignored the most important public health message in the book, "Ah, yes, the quarantine, it didn't do any good."[21]

Or maybe they did understand the limitations of large-scale quarantine but just did not have time to think it through in the post-9/11 panic atmosphere. Lead drafter Gostin, for example, was the group's most articulate critic of quarantine. He told the *Boston Globe* two months after 9/11 that "Not only have quarantines not been effective, they have been the grounds for ignoble responses."[22] And with colleagues at Johns Hopkins, Gostin acknowledged in an article published in *JAMA* in December that quarantines can create more problems than they solve, and "in most infectious disease outbreak scenarios, there are alternatives to large-scale quarantine that may be more medically defensible, more likely to effectively contain the spread of disease, less challenging to implement, and less likely to generate unintended adverse consequences."[23]

Given this, it is remarkable that mass quarantine would be made the centerpiece of public health emergency legislation proposed for the 21st century. As the *JAMA* authors also correctly note, public trust is the key to effective public health action. I wrote an editorial 25 years ago titled "Where Are the Health Lawyers When We Need Them?" arguing that lawyers who work in the medical area "must understand the health care system and how it affects individual patients" if they are to do more good than harm.[24] Today the same message could be brought to lawyers who want to work in the public health and bioterrorism area. For all our sakes, it is critical that fearful public health lawyers not "freak out" and endorse measures that not only violate basic bioethics and human rights principles but also are likely to be counterproductive.

Although they continued to press for adoption of "modernized" state laws, the authors soon conceded that their model act really was more of a "checklist" that states could use to help them decide if changes were needed.[25] In retrospect, it was simply a mistake, perhaps understandably made without careful thought in the immediate aftermath of 9/11. A public that believes that its officials will respect their basic human rights is much more likely to follow reasonable recommendations of public officials in times of emergency. There is no need to trade civil or human rights for safety in this area. In this regard, treating our fellow citizens as the enemy and using police tactics to force treatment and isolate them is much more likely to cost lives than it is to save them. And as a matter of both bioethics and pragmatism, medicine and public health must work *together* to effectively respond to emergencies. Programs that divide Americans and drive their physicians and public health officials apart endanger everyone.

The SARS (severe acute respiratory syndrome) epidemic of 2003 supports these intuitions, and adds another: modern public health must be global in its perspective and actions. No individual country, let alone a state within a country, can effectively deal with a global epidemic alone. The World Health Organization quickly (and appropriately) took the lead in responding to the epidemic by, among other things, initiating travel advisories. Sick people and their physicians and nurses almost universally acted appropriately. Those who were diagnosed with SARS, for example, agreed to voluntary treatment and isolation, and physicians and nurses did not try to avoid their duties (even though they were the ones most at risk of contracting SARS). Public health and medicine were partners, not enemies, in responding to SARS. Finally, mass involuntary quarantines were seldom employed, and where they were, primarily in China, they were ineffective because they produced mistrust of the government that made the epidemic more difficult to deal with. In the United States, no governor declared a state of emergency—so no emergency public health powers were triggered. Instead the public and physicians almost universally cooperated with public health officials, and people who were asked to stay home, in "voluntary quarantine," did so.[26]

Anthrax Vaccine for Civilians

The use of force in public health emergencies is not only unnecessary, it is also most likely to be directed at minorities and the poor, as have quarantines in the past. The lessons from the only actual bioterrorist attack experienced by Americans, the three letters containing anthrax that were sent through the mail in the wake of 9/11, bolster both this observation and the proposition that Americans need accurate information, not intimidation, if we expect Americans to follow public health advice. In these attacks, for example, Americans almost uniformly rushed toward physicians and hospitals (not away from them) and demanded to be screened and treated (rather than resisting such care). Thankfully, even though the initial official government response was antiscientific, public health follow-up was much better, and ultimately only 22 people developed anthrax, 5 of whom died.[27]

More than 10,000 people were advised to take antibiotics on the presumption that they were at risk to contract inhalation anthrax. In late December 2002, the Food and Drug Administration (FDA), DOD, and CDC together released anthrax vaccine that had previously been available only to military personnel for use by those exposed to the anthrax attacks. Of the 10,000 people eligible to take the vaccine, only 152 people actually did.[28] What is the lesson from this experience? Doesn't it, for example, show that it is better to force people to be treated than to leave the decision to individuals?

I think the answer is that although the offer of the anthrax vaccine was extraordinarily clumsy, the CDC and FDA were right to insist that informed consent (the most important doctrine of modern medical ethics) be required and that no one be pressured to take the vaccine. On the other hand, I think they were wrong to make the vaccine available under these highly charged circumstances without making a recommendation to those eligible to take it. If the agencies did not believe that the vaccine was useful as a postexposure treatment, they should not have made it available. If they did believe it was useful, they should have recommended its use and explained the reasons for this recommendation.

To make the vaccine available without a recommendation seems an incredibly cynical political move, designed by the FDA and CDC much more to "cover their respective asses" in case additional people developed anthrax, rather than to help protect those exposed. How else can these two bold-printed lines in the consent form be read?: "DHHS is *not* making any recommendation whether you should or should not take this vaccine. DHHS is making the vaccine available to you to allow you to decide whether or not you wish to use the vaccine."

On what basis (given that there is no data from humans) could individuals make this decision if those with the most experience with the vaccine refused even to advise them about what was medically reasonable? In the context of a government offer to participate in an experiment on a vaccine the government did not recommend, it is easy to understand why at least some black postal workers said they were reminded of Tuskegee and were not about to be made experimental subjects. The legacy of Tuskegee is, of course, one of mistrust in the government, especially in the Public Health Service. Trust, once lost, is extraordinarily difficult to regain, as the Department of Homeland Security has learned from its vague color-coded warnings, and its silly recommendation that Americans stock up on duct tape and plastic sheeting to protect themselves against terrorist attacks.

The flawed process of making the anthrax vaccine available to potentially exposed civilians also raised a generic issue: what should FDA testing rules be for efficacy of drugs and vaccines designed to counteract biological weapons? The FDA has correctly determined that it would be unethical (a violation, for example, of the Nuremberg Code) to conduct human trials of the efficacy of these drugs and vaccines by exposing subjects to potentially lethal agents. But what is the alternative? In 1999 the FDA issued proposed new regulations for comment that suggested that animal testing could substitute for human testing regarding efficacy, and both the U.S. Senate and House of Representatives endorsed this proposed rule in the wake of 9/11. This seems reasonable, and the FDA formally adopted these regulations in 2002.[29] Nonetheless, the fact that these agents, even after they are approved, will not have been tested on humans should mean that their labeling be restricted to "military" or "emergency" use only (no other "unapproved uses"). Moreover, even in emergencies they should only be given when qualified scientists believe them to be the best available alternative, and only with the informed consent of the individuals, soldiers or civilians, involved.

This is one of the lessons from the first Gulf War, when investigational drugs and vaccines were forced on soldiers under the ruse that informed consent was "not feasible." It took an act of Congress to undo the FDA's emergency wartime waiver of informed consent, and we should not make the same mistake again in the war on terror.[30] The mistake was not repeated in the Iraq war, although use of pyridostigmine bromide was approved under the new FDA rules just before the war began.

The administration did, however, make a significant mistake in promoting its program to vaccinate 500,000 health care workers in phase one of a planned three-phase smallpox vaccination project announced in December 2002. Phase two would have encompassed up to 10 million first responders and public safety personnel, and phrase three would have included all willing civilians. Instead of sharing what information was available about the risk of a terrorist attack using smallpox with the American public, the administration relied on double-talk and innuendo. The Director of the CDC, for example, told a U.S. Senate Appropriations Subcommittee on January 29, 2003 (a few months before the start of the Iraq war):

> I can't discuss all of the details because some of the information is, of course, classified. But I think our reading of the intelligence that we share with the intelligence community is that there is a real possibility of a smallpox attack from either nations that are likely to be harboring the virus or from individual entities, such as terrorist cells that could have access to the virus. So we know it's not zero. And I think that's really what we can say with absolute certainty that there is not a zero risk of a smallpox attack.[31]

This marvelous double-talk, of course, proves nothing except that the CDC's director honestly admits that she has no useful knowledge concerning the risks of a smallpox attack. More important, of course, is that if the U.S. government knows that an individual, group, or nation has the smallpox virus and is working to weaponize it, this information should be made public. It is the terrorists who want to keep their methods and intentions secret: the best defense for a potential target is to make this information public. Since most Americans probably know this, the failure of the administration to offer any evidence at all of anyone possessing weaponized smallpox likely meant that the administration had no such evidence. Thus, the real risks of taking the smallpox vaccine could not be offset by any measurable benefit. Accordingly, few were surprised when, with fewer than 40,000 health care workers vaccinated in the first 6 months of the program, it was abandoned as an embarrassing public policy disaster. Informed consent—both to the nation and the individual—really is critical to public trust, which in turn is critical to public health success, even in wartime.[32]

Conclusion

The 9/11 attacks were almost unimaginable, but not totally. Tom Clancy had, in fact, imagined an attack by a hijacked Boeing 747 passenger jet on the U.S. Capitol building in his 1994 novel *Debt of Honor* (although after 9/11 even Clancy said he could never have imagined four planes attacking simultaneously). In Clancy's sequel to *Debt of Honor*, his 1996 *Executive Orders*, he imagines the president declaring a national state of emergency in response to a terrorist attack using a strain of ebola that is transmissible through the air. No expert on law, human rights, or bioethics, Clancy nonetheless makes a point that has escaped many more learned commentators: acts of bioterrorism cannot and will not be dealt with at the state level under the old state "police powers" doctrine. Rather, they are attacks on the United States and will be the responsibility of the federal government under national security powers. Some things have changed irrevocably since 9/11, and one of these is that public health is now (as it should be) a global issue. The SARS epidemic underlined this point. This makes adherence to human rights principles in public health emergencies even more important, because human rights are universal.

In times of war and terror all kinds of overreactions that ignore human rights, including not only consent "waivers" but also proposals for secret trials, unlawful detention, torture, and even misguided "model acts," are predictable. But we cannot prevail by fighting terrorism with terror.

Human rights, especially liberty and democracy, and the U.S. Constitution (not secrecy and unaccountability) are our foundational values. Human rights are not only our ally in war and terror, they are our best defense against aggressors. As Richard Horton, editor of the *Lancet*, eloquently put it less than a month after 9/11:

> Principles of harm reduction are more realistic and practicable than false notions of a war on terrorism. Attacking hunger, disease, poverty, and social exclusion might do more good than air marshals, asylum restrictions, and identity cards. Global security will be achieved only by building stable and strong societies. Health is an undervalued measure of our global security.[33]

We will survive only so long as we uphold human rights. The more we undermine human rights and democracy, the less reason we will have to fight for our survival, and the less we will deserve to survive. In this fight it is critical to recognize that freedom is not just an end of economic development and social justice, it is a means as well.[34] And the importance of human rights (and bioethics) is that they are universal and apply to all humans on the simple basis that we are all members of the same species. It is this recognition, and actions founded on it, that will ultimately preserve both our lives and our liberty. As John F. Kennedy put it so well at American University in the wake of the Cuban missile crisis that came as close as we have ever come to world-destroying nuclear war, in words that were also used to conclude the movie *Thirteen Days*, "no government or social system is so evil that its people must be considered as lacking in virtue." Kennedy continued in reference to the Soviet Union:

> Let us not be blind to our differences—but let us also direct attention to our common interests . . . for in the final analysis, our most common link is that we all inhabit this small planet. We all breathe the same air. We all cherish our children's future. And we are all mortal.

The chief prosecutor at Nuremberg, U.S. Supreme Court Justice Robert Jackson, was, of course, correct to say that "the Constitution is not a suicide pact."[35] But he was more eloquent at Nuremberg when he argued to the judges there that unless we afford all people, even the Nazi defendants, basic human rights, history will rightfully judge us harshly. In his words, "To pass these defendants a poisoned chalice is to put it to our lips as well."[36]

2

. . . .

Human Rights and Health

The modern human rights movement was born from the devastation of World War II.[1] Nonetheless, appeals to universal human rights are at least as old as human government. When Jean Anouilh produced Sophocles's *Antigone* in Nazi-occupied Paris in early 1944, the French audience identified Antigone with the French resistance. Antigone was sentenced to be buried alive for defying King Creon's order not to bury her dead brother (whom the King considered a traitor) but to leave his body to rot in public. The Nazis in the audience also applauded the performance, apparently because they identified with Creon and his difficulty in maintaining law and order in the face of seemingly fanatical resistance.[2]

Antigone, written more than 2400 years ago, focuses on a central moral problem: is there a "higher," universal law to which all humans must answer, or is simply obeying the written law of one's country sufficient? Antigone justified her defiance of the king on the basis of an unwritten, higher law:

> Nor did I think your edict had such force
> that you, a mere mortal, could override the gods,
> the great unwritten, unshakable traditions.

The source of higher law has varied through human history and has included the mythical gods of Olympus, the God of the Old Testament, the God of the New Testament, human reason, and respect for human dignity. The multinational trial of the major Nazi war criminals at Nuremberg following World War II was held on the premise that there is a higher law of humanity (sometimes termed natural law), and that individuals may be properly tried for violating that law. Universal criminal law includes war crimes and crimes against humanity, such as murder, genocide, torture, and slavery. Obeying the orders of superiors is no defense: the state cannot shield its agents from prosecution for crimes against humanity.[3] On December 10, 1948, in a liberated Paris, the nations of the world took another major step toward incorporating human rights into international law by signing the Universal Declaration of Human Rights.

The United Nations (UN) was formed almost immediately after World War II as a permanent peacekeeping organization. The Charter of the United Nations, signed by the 50 original member nations in San Francisco on June 26, 1945, spells out the goals of the United Nations. The first two are: "to save succeeding generations from the scourge of war . . . ; and to reaffirm faith in fundamental human rights, in the dignity and worth of the human person, in the equal rights of men and women and of nations large and small." After the charter was signed, the adoption of an international bill of rights with legal authority proceeded in three steps: a declaration, two treaties, and implementation measures.

The Universal Declaration of Human Rights

The Universal Declaration of Human Rights was adopted by the UN General Assembly in 1948 without dissent, 48 member states voting in favor and eight abstaining (Saudi Arabia, South Africa, and the Soviet Union together with five other votes it controlled) as a "common standard for all peoples and nations."[4] As Henry Steiner notes, "No other document has so caught the historical moment, achieved the same moral and rhetorical force, or exerted so much influence on the human rights movement as a whole."[5] The rights spelled out in the declaration "stem from the cardinal axiom that all human beings are born free and equal, in dignity and rights, and are endowed with reason and conscience. All the rights and freedoms belong to everybody. . . ."[6] Of special importance to health care professionals and bioethicists is Article 25, which provides in part that "Everyone has the right to a standard of living adequate for the health and well-being of himself and his family, including food, clothing, housing and medical care and necessary social services. . . ." The document is reprinted in Appendix A.

Unlike ethical precepts that primarily govern individual conduct, human rights are primarily rights individuals have against governments. Human rights require governments to respect human rights by refraining from doing certain things, such as torture and limiting freedom of religion, to protect human rights, and also to fulfill human rights by taking actions to make people's lives better such as providing education and nutrition programs. The United Nations adopted the Universal Declaration of Human Rights as a statement of aspirations. Legal obligations of governments were to derive from formal treaties that member nations would individually sign and incorporate into their domestic law.

The Treaties

Because of the cold war, with its conflicting governmental ideologies, it took almost 20 years to achieve agreement on the texts of the two major human rights treaties. The International Covenant on Civil and Political Rights (reprinted in Appendix B), and the International Covenant on Economic, Social, and Cultural Rights (reprinted in Appendix C) were both adopted by the UN General Assembly and opened for signature and ratification on December 16, 1966. The United States ratified the International Covenant on Civil and Political Rights in 1992, but not surprisingly, given our capitalist economic system with its emphasis on private property, has yet to act on the International Covenant on Economic, Social, and Cultural Rights. The division of human rights into two separate treaties illustrates the worldwide tension between the tradition of liberal states founded on civil and political rights and socialist and communist welfare states founded on solidarity and the government's obligation to provide for basic human needs.

The rights spelled out in the International Covenant on Civil and Political Rights include equality, the right to liberty and security of person, and freedom of movement, religion, expression, and association. The International Covenant on Economic, Social, and Cultural Rights focuses on human well-being, including the right to work; the right to fair wages, a decent living, and safe and healthy working conditions; the right to be free from hunger; the right to education; and "the right of everyone to the enjoyment of the highest attainable standard of physical and mental health."

Given the horrors of poverty, disease, and wars since World War II, it is easy to dismiss the rights enunciated in these documents as empty gestures. Amnesty International, for example, in marking the 50th anniversary of the Universal Declaration of Human Rights, labeled the rights it articulates "little more than a paper promise" for most people in the world.[7] Amnesty is certainly correct that unadulterated celebration is not in order, but as Joseph Kunz noted more than 50 years ago in writing about the birth of the Universal Declaration of Human Rights, "In the field of human rights as in other actual problems of international law it is necessary to avoid the Scylla of a pessimistic cynicism and the Charybdis of mere wishful thinking and superficial optimism."[8]

Human Rights and Health

The Universal Declaration of Human Rights and the two subsequent treaties form a global human rights framework for action and have a special relevance for global health. The relationship between health and human rights has been most persuasively articulated and most tirelessly championed by Jonathan Mann, the first director of the World Health Organization's (WHO) Global Programme on AIDS, whose life was tragically cut short in the 1998 crash of Swissair flight 111. The strongest predictive indicator of health is income, which is another way to say that poverty has a strong correlation with disease and disability, and one way to attack disease and improve health internationally is to redistribute income.[9] This seems a hopeless goal to most people in the developing nations, and reliance on income redistribution as a single or primary strategy can create a sense of disabling pessimism that nothing can be done, or cynicism that nothing will be done.[10] Income equality is unattainable. But it is not unreasonable to expect the richer nations to share their wealth with the poorer nations and to thereby help create the conditions necessary for good health for all. The United Nations has noted, for example, that the cost of universal access to basic education, health care, food, and clean water is as little as $40 billion a year—less than four percent of the combined wealth of the 225 richest people in the world.[11] This figure seems too low (if two billion people need additional resources, it would provide only $20 each). Nonetheless, it focuses on proper global goals and makes the valid point that not much redistribution would be required to have a major impact on the lives of most people in the world.

Multinational corporations must become actively involved in promoting human rights as well, because they control much of the wealth of the planet. This has become evident in the global environmental movement in the areas of pollution, resource conservation, and global warming and should be evident in health care as well. Much of the research agenda on drugs and vaccines, for example, is controlled by large multinational pharmaceutical corporations, not by governments.

By broadening our perspective, human rights language highlights basic human needs such as equality, education, nutrition, and sanitation, whose improvement will have a major impact on improving human health. Before the WHO became more active at the turn of the century, international leadership in world health in the 1990s centered in the World Bank. In 1993 the World Bank issued a report titled *Investing in Health*.[12] Although not stated in the language of human rights, the report's action agenda implicitly acknowledged that only the recognition of basic human rights could improve the health status of most of the world's population. In developing countries, for example, the World Bank's two primary recommendations for improvement of health were "increased investment in schooling for girls" and the financing of a basic package of public health programs, including AIDS prevention. The other major recommendations included increasing the income of the poor, promoting the rights and status of women through "political and economic empowerment and legal protection against abuse," and delivering essential clinical services to the poor. These recommendations directly address the human rights issues of access to education, access to health care, and discrimination against women. Ten years later, in 2003, the World Bank issued a report on the effects of war on development, specifically on the 52 major civil wars that were fought from 1960 to 1999. The report, *Breaking the Conflict Trap: Civil War and Development Policy*, not surprisingly concluded that civil war leaves a country in persistent poverty and with a high level of disease.[13] Wars, both global and local, were a persistent theme of the past century and have so far continued unabated into the 21st century. No public health program can prevent disease and death in a world dedicated to violence.

Human Rights and Public Health

World War II, arguably the first truly global war, led to a global acknowledgment of the universality of human rights and the responsibility of governments to promote them. Jonathan Mann perceptively noted that the AIDS epidemic can be viewed as the first global epidemic because it is taking place at a time when all countries are linked both electronically and by swift transportation.[14] Like World War II, this worldwide tragedy requires us to think in new ways and to develop effective methods to treat and prevent disease on a global level. Globalization is a mercantile and ecological fact; it is also becoming a health care reality. The challenge facing medicine and health care is to develop a global language and a global strategy that can help to improve the health of all of the world's citizens. Clinical medicine is practiced one patient at a time, and the language of medical ethics is the language of self-determination and beneficence: doing what is in the best interests of the patient with the patient's informed consent. This is powerful but has little direct application in countries where physicians are scarce and medical resources very limited.

Public health deals with populations and prevention—the necessary frame of reference in the global context. In a one-to-one doctor–patient relationship, for example, a combination of antiretroviral drugs for AIDS treatment makes sense. In the worldwide pandemic, however, such treatment may be available to fewer than five percent of the world's people with AIDS.[15] This is not just a matter of money but also a matter of health care infrastructure and a lack of basic knowledge regarding how to effectively deliver drugs. These issues are addressed in Chapter 5 in the context of nevirapine for pregnant women in South Africa. In dealing with the AIDS pandemic it has become necessary to deal directly with issues of discrimination, immigration status, the rights of women, privacy, and informed consent as well as education and access to health care. Although it is easy to recognize that population-based prevention is required to effectively address the AIDS epidemic on a global level (as well as, for example, tuberculosis, malaria, and tobacco-related illness), it has been much harder to articulate a global public health ethic, and public health itself has had an extraordinarily difficult time developing its own ethical language.[16] Because of its universality and its emphasis on equality and dignity, the language of human rights is well suited for public health.

On the occasion of the 50th anniversary of the Universal Declaration of Human Rights, I suggested that the declaration itself sets forth the ethics of public health, given that its goal is to provide the conditions under which humans can flourish.[17] This is also the goal of public health, making it reasonable for public health to adopt the Universal Declaration of Human Rights as its code of ethics. The unification of public health and human rights workers around the globe would be a powerful force to improve the lives of everyone. Without, I think, being seduced into the wishful thinking category, it should be stressed that the Universal Declaration of Human Rights is a much more powerful health document than it was in 1948 because both our global interdependence and human equality are better recognized today.

Human Rights and Physicians

Both medical ethics and human rights are aspirational and difficult to enforce. Over the past two decades American medical ethics has been de
facto transformed into medical law, with more litigation and enforcement
and the increasing marginalization of aspirational ethics.[18] Moreover, the
much broader field of bioethics has yet to live up to its promise to incorporate planetary concerns, such as ecology, into its agenda. American bioethics seems to be shrinking, as most recently illustrated by its fixation with
embryonic stem cell research. The human rights field, on the other hand,
is growing. Cynicism is understandable, given the use of rights rhetoric to
justify tyrannical acts. Nonetheless, human rights remains the standard, and
gross human rights abuses, such as those at Abu Ghraib prison, cannot be
publicly condoned. Not only are human rights being taken more seriously
by governments, but they are also increasingly a major driving force in
private, nongovernmental organizations (NGOs). Of course, there are different kinds of rights and more or less effective ways to enforce them. The
new International Criminal Court can, for example, help to deter and punish
those who engage in torture and genocide but can do nothing to governments that fail to provide basic health care to their citizens. Moreover, to
conclude that human rights is a much more powerful language for good
than is medical ethics is not to conclude that medical ethics is irrelevant.
On the contrary, medical ethics not only is necessary to make basic human
rights a reality (for example, by prohibiting physician involvement in torture and executions), but also can advance an antipaternalistic public health
agenda that supports public education and democracy in public health
practice. It thus seems more fruitful to explore the ways in which bioethics
and human rights act symbiotically than to ignore either (or both) of them.

Individuals and NGOs can use human rights language and concepts
to inspire and energize their own activities. Many physician groups have
been leaders in promoting human rights, including International Physicians
for the Prevention of Nuclear War (IPPNW) and its U.S. affiliate Physicians
for Social Responsibility (PSR), Physicians for Human Rights (PHR),
Médecins sans Frontières (Doctors without Borders), and Médecins du
Monde (Doctors of the World). Global Lawyers and Physicians (GLP)
broadens the base by providing an opportunity for physicians and lawyers
to work together to promote human rights and health. Physicians and other
health care professionals interested in promoting human rights thus have
many organizations they can support, most of which have concentrated
primarily on the medical and health disasters created by wars, torture, abuses

of prisoners, and arbitrary detention as well as the threats to health created by nuclear, chemical, and biological weapons, land mines, and other means of killing and maiming.

The fact that the Universal Declaration of Human Rights itself is a declaration, not a treaty, need not limit its reach any more than that fact failed to limit the reach of the Declaration of Independence. Although the Declaration of Independence started a war and the Universal Declaration of Human Rights was drafted to prevent war, it is the power of its concepts and language that matter most. As has been properly noted, the U.S. Declaration of Independence "rests less in law than in the minds and hearts of the people, and its meaning changes as new groups and new causes claim its mantle."[19] Lincoln, for example, claimed to be upholding the "all men are created equal" pronouncement of the declaration when he spoke at Gettysburg and when he issued the Emancipation Proclamation. And a century later, Martin Luther King, Jr., stood at the site of the Lincoln Memorial and invoked the words of the declaration in calling for a new birth of the freedom Lincoln had promised, by which he meant "an end to the poverty, discrimination, and segregation that left black citizens 'languishing in the corners of American society,' exiles in their own land."[20]

The meaning of the Universal Declaration of Human Rights for the world's citizens will be similarly invoked and reinterpreted to meet the changing challenges of the times. For example, the agendas of all of those who support human rights should be broad, including efforts to make basic health care available to all who need it, to prevent disease and injury, and to promote health worldwide.

It took more than 2000 years for the Antigone-type appeal to a higher law to justify defiance of government decrees to mature into an international declaration of universal rights. In only slightly more than 50 years after the promulgation of the Universal Declaration of Human Rights, human rights language pervades international politics, law, and morality. The challenge now is to make the promise of the Universal Declaration of Human Rights a reality. In meeting this challenge, American bioethics is a critical consort.

3

. . . .

The Man on the Moon

G enetics has been not only the most superheated scientific arena of the past decade, it has also been a feverish battlefield for American bioethics. And no area has elicited as much controversy as the speculative prospect of genetic engineering—the subject of this and the next chapter.[1] We cannot know what human life will be like a thousand years from now, but we can and should think seriously about what we would like it to be like. What is unique about human beings and about being human; what makes humans human? What qualities of the human species must we preserve to preserve humanity itself? What would a "better human" be like? If genetic engineering techniques work, are there human qualities we should try to temper and others we should try to enhance? If human rights and human dignity depend on our human nature, can we change our "humanness" without undermining our dignity and our rights? At the outset of the third millennium, we can begin our exploration of these questions by looking back on some of the major events and themes of the past 1000 years in Western civilization and the primitive human instincts they illustrate.

Holy Wars

The second millennium opened with holy wars: local wars, such as the Spanish Reconquista to retake Spain from the Moors, and the broader multistate Crusades to take the Holy Lands from the Muslims, who were menacing Christian pilgrims there. The great Crusades, which lasted almost 200 years, were fought in the name of God, with the war cry *Deus volt* ("God wills it").[2] The enemy was the nonbeliever, the infidel, and killing the infidel became a holy act. The ability to label an enemy as "other" and subhuman and to justify killing the other for the sake of God (or country) was to become the primary recurring theme of the entire millennium. Both the Reconquista and the Crusades reverberated in 3/11, the al Qaeda train-bombing massacre in Madrid.

Like the crusaders, Columbus sought to conquer new territories peopled by infidels in the name of God. When Columbus reached the "new" world, which he mistakenly thought was part of India, he named the island on which he landed San Salvador and claimed it in the name of the Catholic Church and the Catholic monarchs of Spain.[3] Naming for Europeans was emblematic of conquest, of taking possession, and could be symbolized with a flag. But Columbus, whose professed goal was also to convert the "savages" who inhabited the new world, is recorded as saying, "in all regions I always left a cross standing" as a mark of Christian dominance.[4] Religion was the cover story for the conquest. Nonetheless, Columbus's encounter with the Native Americans, or "Indians," resulted in their merciless subjugation and genocidal destruction.[5]

The Spanish conquistadors who followed Columbus continued to use the Catholic religion and its absence in the New World as an excuse to claim the land and conquer the inhabitants. In his *The History of the Conquest of Mexico*, for example, William Prescott recounts the European belief that paganism was to be regarded "as a sin to be punished with fire . . . in this world, and eternal suffering in the next." Prescott continues, "Under this code, the territory of the heathen, wherever found [was forfeit to the Holy See] and as such was freely given away by the head of the Church to any temporal potentate whom he pleased that would assume the burden of conquest." Prescott seems to have had some sympathy for Montezuma (the sun god) and the other Aztecs killed by the Spaniards in their conquest, but he ultimately concludes that the Aztecs did not deserve to be considered fully human: "How can a nation, where human sacrifices prevail, and especially when combined with cannibalism, further the march of civilization?"[6]

In similar fashion, Pizarro justified his conquest of Peru and the subjugation of the Incas, including the kidnapping and killing of Atahuallpa, by claiming it was for the "glory of God" and to bring "to our holy Catholic faith so vast a number of heathens." Although God was the cover story, the real motive was gold. In pursuing El Dorado, the city of gold, none of the Spanish conquistadors who followed Cortés and Pizarro (who extracted the world's largest ransom in gold for Atahuallpa) were, however, able to plunder the amount of gold they did.

The Crusades, the voyages of Columbus, and the slaughters by the Spanish conquistadors who followed are powerful metaphors for human exploration and human encounters with the unknown. They teach us that the realm of human dominance can be radically enlarged by human imagination and courage. More importantly, they teach us that without a belief in human dignity and equality, the cost of such dominance is genocidal human rights violations. They also caution us to be suspicious of stated motives and cover stories: although filled with missionary zeal, most of these adventurers and explorers sought primarily fame and fortune.

Unholy Wars

It is, of course, much easier to look back 500 years than 50 years. Nonetheless, World War II, the Apollo moon landings, and the prospect of human genetic engineering raise most of the important issues we face in the new millennium in defining humanness, human rights, and science's responsibilities. Postmodernism can be dated from any of these, and each holds its own lessons and cautions. Many scholars date postmodernism from Hiroshima and the Holocaust, one an instantaneous annihilation, the other a systematic one.[7] Together, their application of industrial techniques to human slaughter represents the death of our civilization's dream of moral and scientific progress that had characterized the modern age. The nuclear age is much more ambiguous and uncertain. We now worship science as society's new religion as the quest for everlasting life with God is replaced by our new crusade for immortality on earth.

As discussed in the previous chapter, the modern human rights movement was born from the blood of World War II and the death of the positive law belief that the only law that matters is that which is enacted by a legitimate government, including the Nazi government. The multinational trial of the Nazi war criminals at Nuremberg after World War II was held on the premise that there is a universal law of humanity and that those who violate it may be properly tried and punished. Universal criminal law, law that applies to all humans and protects all humans, outlaws crimes against humanity, including state-sanctioned genocide, murder, torture, and slavery.

Obeying the laws of a particular country or the orders of superiors is no defense.[8]

The crusades were also echoed in World War II. General Dwight Eisenhower titled his account of World War II *Crusade in Europe*, and his order of the day for the D-Day invasion read: "Soldiers, sailors, and airmen of the allied expeditionary forces, you are about to embark on a great crusade . . . the hopes and prayers of liberty loving people everywhere march with you." And as with the crusades and the conquest of the Americas, to justify the human slaughter of World War II the enemy had to be dehumanized. On the Allied side, the most dehumanizing language was meted out to the Japanese:

> Among the Allies the Japanese were also known as "jackals"' or "monkey men" or "sub-humans," the term of course used by the Germans for Russians, Poles, and assorted Slavs, amply justifying their vivisection . . . *Jap* . . . was a brisk monosyllable handy for slogans like "Rap the Jap" or "Let's Blast the Jap Clean Off the Map," the last a virtual prophecy of Hiroshima.[9]

The United Nations was formed to prevent further wars and on the premise that *all* humans have dignity and are entitled to equal rights. Science and medicine came under specific investigation in the 1946–47 "Doctors' Trial" of 23 Nazi physician-experimenters.[10] The Nazi experiments involved murder and torture, systematic and barbarous acts with death as the planned endpoint. The subjects of these experiments, which included lethal freezing and high-altitude experiments, were concentration camp prisoners, mostly Jews, Gypsies, and Slavs, people the Nazis viewed as subhuman. With echoes of the conquest of the Americas, Nazi philosophy was founded on the belief that Germans were a "superior race" whose destiny was to subjugate and rule the inferior races.[11] A central part of the Nazi project was eugenics, the attempt to improve the species, mostly by eliminating "inferior" people, so-called useless eaters.[12] In its final judgment, the court articulated what we now know as the Nuremberg Code. This code, which is reproduced in Appendix D, remains the most authoritative legal and ethical document governing international research standards and requires the informed consent of every research subject. It is one of the premier human rights documents in world history, and the primary contribution of American bioethics to the international community to date.

The trials at Nuremberg were soon followed by the adoption of the Universal Declaration of Human Rights in 1948, which is, as previously discussed, the most important human rights document to date. This was followed by two treaties, the Covenant on Civil and Political Rights and the Covenant on Economic, Social, and Cultural Rights. The Universal Declaration of Human Rights and the two treaties represent a milestone for humanity: the recognition that human rights are founded on human dignity and that human dignity is shared by *all* members of the human race without distinctions based on race, religion, or national origin.[13]

The Man on the Moon

The most spectacular exploration of the 20th century was the voyage of Apollo 11 to the moon's surface and the safe return of its crew. Neil Armstrong's words upon setting foot on the moon seemed just right: "One small step for [a] man, one giant leap for mankind [*sic*]." Although the race to the moon had more to do with the politics of the cold war than science, it was nonetheless an almost magical engineering accomplishment.[14] And, like Columbus, history will remember Armstrong because he was the first to set foot on the moon.

The United States was willing to go to great lengths to ensure that the first man on the moon would be American and would plant an American flag on the moon. Nonetheless, there were human rights constraints even on this experiment. President John Kennedy, for example, had set it as a United States goal to land a man on the moon "and return him safely to earth." Putting human values second to winning a race with the Russians by landing a man on the moon without a clear plan for getting him back to Earth was rejected.

The United States did not explicitly conquer the moon for the glory of God, but God was on the minds of the conquerors riding in a spacecraft named for the sun god, Apollo. Some of the most explicit religious statements were made by rocket designer Werner Von Braun, who had been a Nazi SS officer and the designer of the destructive V2 rockets that the Germans rained down on England near the end of World War II. Von Braun was captured by the United States and "sanitized" to work on rocket propulsion, eventually heading up NASA's effort. The day before Apollo 11 blasted off he explained the reasons for putting a man on the moon: "We are expanding the mind of man. We are extending this God-given brain and these God-given hands to their outermost limits and in so doing all mankind will benefit. All mankind will reap the harvest. . . ."[15] The missionary zeal of the Crusaders and conquistadors was to echo on the moon.

Norman Mailer, in his chronicle of the moon landing *Of a Fire on the Moon*, asks a central question: "Was the voyage of Apollo 11 the noblest expression of the technological age, or the best evidence of its utter insanity? . . . are we witness to grandeur or madness?"[16] Today neither extreme seems quite right. The moon rocks returned to earth were only a poor symbol of the trip, but the photos of Earth taken from space have had a profound impact on our global consciousness, if not our global conscience, and have helped energize the worldwide environmental protection movement. It is much harder to deny our common humanity when we can all see our common home.

We now know that the Russians were never serious challengers in the moon race and that the prospect of the United States following the moon landing with a serious effort at space exploration was grossly overstated. Our loss of enchantment, even interest, in the moon was captured by Gene Cernam, the last of the 12 astronauts to land on the moon, when he said, as he blasted off its surface, "Let's get this mother out of here."[17] The moon landing was primarily about commerce and politics, not peace and harmony. As historian Walter McDougall notes in his book *The Heavens and the Earth,* although the plaque we placed on the moon read "We came in peace for all mankind," peace was not what the mission was about. It did have something to do with science and national pride, but he argues, "mostly it was about spy satellites and comsats and other orbital systems for military and commercial advantage."[18] Military and commercial goals continue to dominate outer space, just as they did with the conquistadors. And even though manned space exploration has again been relegated to the realm of science fiction, the moon landing continues to be the scientific and engineering feat to which those aspiring to breakthrough innovation compare their efforts.

It is in the realm of science fiction that most of the important speculation about the human predicament and the future of humanity is envisioned. It was Jorge Luis Borges, for example, who first suggested that humans could become immortal if they were willing to have all of their bodily functions performed by machines. Humans could enter into the world of pure thought by having their brains inhabit a "cube-like" piece of furniture. In the nightmare envisioned by Borges, modern surgery and mechanical replacement parts could bring a type of immortality to humankind, not as immortal actors, but as immortal witnesses.[19]

Arthur Clarke, in *2001: A Space Odyssey*, suggests that human evolution might move in a different direction: toward the development of a computerized mind encapsulated in a metal spaceshiplike body, eternally roaming the galaxy in search of new sensations.[20] The price for human immortality in this view is the eradication of both the human body and the human mind, the former being replaced by an artificial, destruction-proof container, the latter by an infinitely replicable computer program. Of course, the indestructible robot body inhabited by a digitalized memory chip would not be human in the sense we understand it today, and the rights of this assemblage would likely be more on the order of the rights of robots than those of contemporary humans.

We could use our technology to explore outer space with such robots, but our current fascination is focused on inner space. Instead of expanding our minds and our perspectives as a species by pondering the mysteries of outer space with its possibilities of other life forms, we are turning inward and contemplating ourselves on the microscopic level. The new biology, perhaps better described as the new genetics or the "genetics age," suggests a biology-based immortality alternative to a digital brain in a body of metal and plastic: changing and "enhancing" our human capabilities by altering our genes at the molecular level. Or, as James Watson, the codiscoverer of the structure of DNA, famously put it, "We used to think our future was in our stars, now we know our future is in our genes."[21]

Genetic Engineering

Like space exploration, work on human genetics is dominated by governmental agencies and commercial interests. Taking place in the shadow of Hiroshima and under the ever-present threat of species suicide by nuclear annihilation, genetics research can be seen as an attempt by science to redeem itself, to bring the "gift" of immortality to a species whose very existence it has placed at risk.[22] The scientific (and commercial) goal is unabashedly to conquer death by engineering the immortal human. As the head of Human Genome Sciences declared, "Death is a series of preventable diseases."[23] Basic strategies to construct a "better human" are suggested by two genetic experiments: cloning sheep and making a smarter mouse.

In 1997 embryologist Ian Wilmut announced that he and his colleagues had cloned a sheep, creating a genetic twin of an adult animal by reprogramming one of its somatic cells to act as the nucleus of an enucleated egg.[24] He called the cloned lamb Dolly. An international debate on outlawing the cloning of a human began immediately and has continued. Dolly's "creator," Wilmut, has consistently argued that his cloning technique should not be applied to humans for reproduction.[25] He has not used literature to bolster his argument, but he could.

One reporter who described Wilmut as "Dolly's laboratory father," for example, could not have conjured up images of Mary Shelley's *Frankenstein* better if he had tried. Frankenstein was also his creature's father–god; the creature tells him: "I ought to be thy Adam." Like Dolly, the "spark of life" was infused into the creature by electric current. Unlike Dolly, Frankenstein's creature was created fully grown (not a cloning possibility) and wanted more than creaturehood. He wanted a mate of his "own kind" with whom to live and reproduce. Frankenstein reluctantly agreed to manufacture such a mate if the creature agreed to leave humankind alone. But in the end Frankenstein viciously destroys the female creature–mate, concluding that he has no right to inflict the children of this pair, "a race of devils," upon "everlasting generations." Frankenstein ultimately recognized his responsibility to humanity, and Shelley's great novel explores almost all the noncommercial elements of today's cloning debate.[26]

The naming of the world's first cloned mammal, like the naming of San Salvador and the Apollo spacecraft, is telling. The sole survivor of 277 cloned embryos (or "fused couplets"), the clone could have been named after its sequence in this group (for example, 6LL3), but this would have only emphasized its character as a product. In stark contrast, the name Dolly suggests a unique individual. Victor Frankenstein, of course, never named his creature, thereby repudiating any parental responsibility. By naming the world's first mammal clone Dolly, Wilmut accepted responsibility for her.

Cloning is replication and as such holds little attraction or interest for people who want to have children. Most of us want our children to have better lives than we have had, not simply to duplicate ours, even genetically. That is why genetic engineering experiments that promise "better" children (and better humans) are much more important to the future of humankind. In 1999, for example, Princeton scientist Joe Tsien announced that he had used genetic engineering techniques to create mice that had better memories and could therefore learn faster than other mice; they were "smarter."[27] Tsien is convinced that if his findings can be made applicable to humans, everyone will want to use genetic engineering to have smarter babies. In his words, "Everyone wants to be smart."

Appropriating the moon landing metaphor, Tsien said of his genetically engineered mice (he named the strain Doogie after TV's fictional boy genius physician), "To the scientific community this is a small step for a man. The fundamental question is, 'Is this a giant step for mankind?'"[28] Tsien has also suggested that his work is much more important than cloning because a genetic duplicate adds nothing new to the world. His point is well taken. The possibility of applying genetic engineering techniques to humans for the purpose of making smarter, stronger, happier, prettier, or longer-lived humans simultaneously raises all the questions I posed at the beginning of this chapter: what does it mean to be human, and what changes in "humanness" would result in better humans (or a new species altogether)?

In the world of genetic engineering, our children would become products of our own manufacture.[29] As products, they would be subject to both quality control and improvements, including destruction and replacement if they were "defective." We could construct a new eugenics based not on a corrupt, Hitlerean view of our fellow humans, but on a utopian dream of what an ideal child should be like. Do we really want what we seem to want? Is Tsien correct, for example, in claiming that everyone would want to have a better memory?

Elie Wiesel, the most eloquent witness of the Holocaust, has devoted his life's work to memory, trying to ensure that the world cannot forget the horrors of the Holocaust so that they won't be repeated.[30] This was also the primary aim of the prosecution and judges at the International Military Tribunal at Nuremberg. The crimes against humanity committed during World War II had to be remembered. As chief prosecutor Justice Robert Jackson put it to the tribunal, "The wrongs which we seek to condemn and punish have been so calculated, so malignant, and so devastating, that civilization cannot tolerate their being ignored because it cannot survive their being repeated." It is obviously not just memory itself that matters, but the information memory holds and what humans do with that information. We have, for example, more and more information about our genes every day. We are told that scientists will soon be able to understand life at the molecular level. But in pursuing this objective we have lost all perspective. We do not live life on the molecular level, but as full persons. We will never be able to understand life (or how it should be lived, or what it means to be human) by exploring or understanding our lives or our bodies at the molecular, atomic, or even the subatomic level.[31]

Cloned sheep live in a pen, and laboratory mice are confined in a controlled environment. Science now seems to act as if humanity's goal is a world of mass contentment and containment, an earth-sized human zoo in which every man, woman, and child has all the "smart genes" we can provide, is fed the most nutritious food, is protected from all preventable diseases, lives in a clean, air-filtered environment, and is supplied sufficient mind-altering drugs to be in a constant state of happiness, even euphoria. And this happy life, which Borges envisioned with horror, could be made to extend for hundreds of years, at least if there is no more to life than a perfectly engineered body, a contented mind, and virtual immortality. Bio-ethicist Leon Kass has put it well in the context of genetic engineering (but he could also have been speaking of Columbus): "Though well-equipped, we know not who we are or where we are going."[32] We literally don't know what to make of ourselves. Humans must inform science; science cannot inform (or define) humanity. Novelty is not progress, and technique cannot substitute for life's meaning and purpose.

Toward the Posthuman

As we attempt to take human evolution into our own hands, it is not the Aztecs or the Nazis whom we next plan to conquer. The territory we now claim is our own body. We claim it in the name of the new eugenic right of every human to do with his or her body what he or she chooses. Yet the brief history of our species cautions that there are limits to both our knowl-edge and our claims of dominion. Cortés could rationalize his subjugation of the Aztecs because, among other things, they engaged in human sacri-fice and cannibalism. With human experimentation, such as the transplan-tation of a heart from a baboon to Baby Fae, we have made human sacrifice an art (albeit in the name of science rather than God), and with organ trans-plantation we have tamed cannibalism.[33] Postmodern man accepts no lim-its, no taboos.

If humanity survives another 1000 years, what will the human of the year 3000 be like? With more than three-quarters of Earth covered by water, would the addition of gills, for example, be an enhancement or a defor-mity?[34] Would a child be reared with gills for underwater exploration or for a circus sideshow?[35] How tall is too tall? Can you be too smart for your own good? If we continue to ignore the continuing pollution of our envi-ronment, perhaps the improved human should be able to breathe polluted air and survive on garbage. As we deplete our energy sources, perhaps the improved human should have a bionic wheel to replace our legs for more efficient mobility. Or perhaps we should try to grow wings to fly. Will we as a society permit individual scientists to try any or all of these experi-ments on humans, or can we learn from the unanticipated consequences of conquest and war that humans are better off when they think before they act, and act democratically when action can have a profound impact on every member of our species?

It was to prevent war that the United Nations was formed, and it was to hold people accountable for crimes against humanity, such as murder, torture, slavery, and genocide, that the International Criminal Court was established. Of course, state-sponsored crimes against humanity are still committed. But the world no longer ignores the rights of peoples who earlier in the century would simply have been designated "uncivilized" or considered subhuman.[36] If we humans are to be the masters of our own destiny and not simply products of our new technologies (a big "if"), we will need to build international institutions sturdier than the United Nations and the International Criminal Court to help channel and control our newfound powers and to protect basic human rights. Human dignity and equality are only likely to be safe if science is accountable to democratic institutions and transparent enough that international deliberation can take place before irrevocable species-endangering experiments are conducted.

Outside the realm of creating and producing weapons of mass destruction, science is not a criminal activity, and human cloning and genetic engineering do not "fit" comfortably in the category of crimes against humanity. Moreover, in the face of the Holocaust and nuclear weapons, genetic engineering appears almost benign. But this is deceptive because genetic engineering has the capacity to change the meaning of what it is to be human. There are limits to how far we can go in changing our nature without changing our humanity and our basic human values. Because it is the meaning of humanness (our distinctness from other animals) that has given birth to our concepts of both human dignity and human rights, altering our nature threatens to undermine our concepts of both human dignity and human rights. With their loss the fundamental belief in human equality would also be lost. Of course, we know that the rich are much better off than the poor and that real equality will require income redistribution. Nonetheless, the rich may not enslave, torture, or kill even the poorest human on the planet. Likewise, it is a fundamental premise of democracy that all humans, even the poor, must have a voice in determining the future of our species and our planet.

Can universal human rights and democracy, grounded on human dignity, survive human genetic engineering? Without clear goals, the market will define what a better human is. Mass marketing and advertising will encourage us to conform to some culturally constructed ideal rather than celebrate differences. This is at least one major lesson learned from the cosmetic surgery industry: almost all of its patient–clients want either to be reconstructed to appear normal or to be remodeled to appear younger.[37] It should at least give an immortality-seeking science (and society) pause that the more the human life span has increased, the more human societies devalue and marginalize the aged and idolize and seek to emulate the bodies of the young.

The new ideal human, the genetically engineered "superior" human, will almost certainly come to represent "the other."[38] If history is a guide, either the normal humans will view the "better" humans as the other and seek to control or destroy them, or vice-versa. The better human will become, at least in the absence of a universal concept of human dignity, either the oppressor or the oppressed. In short, as H. G. Wells made clear in his *Valley of the Blind*, it is simply untrue that every "enhancement" of human ability will be universally praised: in the valley of the blind, eyes that functioned were considered a deformity to be surgically eliminated so that the sighted person would be like everyone else.[39] In *The Time Machine* Wells himself envisioned the division of humans into two separate and hostile species, neither any improvement over existing humans.[40]

Ultimately, it is almost inevitable that genetic engineering will move *Homo sapiens* to develop into two separable species: the standard-issue human beings will be like the savages of the pre-Columbian Americas and be seen by the new genetically enhanced posthumans as heathens who can properly be slaughtered and subjugated. It is this genocidal potential that makes some species-altering genetic engineering projects potential species-endangering weapons of mass destruction, and the unaccountable genetic engineer a potential bioterrorist. Science cannot save us from our inhumanity toward one another, it can just make our destructive tendencies more efficient and more bestial. Science and oppression can, in fact, go hand in hand. As historian Robert Proctor put it in concluding his study of public health under the Third Reich, "the routine practice of science can so easily coexist with routine exercise of cruelty."[41]

New Crusades

Although we humans have not conquered death, we have invented an immortal creature: the corporation. The corporation is a legal fiction endowed by law with eternal life (and limited liability). This creature has, like Frankenstein's monster, assumed powers not envisioned or controllable by its creator. In its contemporary form, the corporation has become transnational and thus under the control of no government, democratic or otherwise. It swears no allegiance to anything and knows no limits in its pursuit of growth and profit. And as did the Spanish Crown, it has its own cover story. Corporations, at least life sciences and biotechnology corporations, seek profits not for their own sake, according to their cover stories, but rather do scientific research for the betterment of mankind. Some in the life sciences corporate world now seek to make not only better plants and animals, but also better humans. Orwell's *Animal Farm*, where "all animals are equal, but some are more equal than others," now seems much more likely to be brought to us by life sciences corporations than by totalitarian dictatorships. Science fiction writer Michael Crichton first seemed to notice that "the commercialization of molecular biology is the most stunning ethical event in the history of science, and it has happened with astonishing speed."[42]

Science's crusade no longer seeks eternal life with God, but eternal life on earth. In decoding the human genome, religion is again the cover story, as scientists speak of the genome as the "book of man" [*sic*] and the "holy grail" of biology. But it is still gold and glory that these modern-day, corporation-sponsored explorers seek. Because there is money to be made by doing it, the corporate redesign of humans is inevitable in the absence of what Vaclav Havel has termed "a transformation of the spirit and the human relationship to life and the world." Havel has noted that the new "dictatorship of money" has replaced totalitarianism, but it is equally capable of sapping life of its meaning with its "materialistic obsessions," the "flourishing of selfishness," and its need "to evade personal responsibility." Without responsibility our future is bleak. Like the failed quest of the Spanish conquistadors for El Dorado, our quest for more and more money will fizzle. Immortality without purpose is also hollow. In Havel's words, "the only kind of politics that makes sense is a politics that grows out of the imperative, and the need, to live as everyone ought to live and therefore—to put it somewhat dramatically—to bear responsibility for the entire world."[43]

To bear responsibility for the entire world may seem excessive, but even Frankenstein would recognize it as just right. It reminds us of the environmental movement's mantra "think globally, act locally" and makes each of us responsible for all of us. How can we, citizens of the world, regain some control over science and industry that threatens to alter our species and the very meaning of our lives? It will not be easy, and given the consistently brutish nature of our species, perhaps we do not deserve to survive. Nonetheless, the worldwide rejection of the prospect of cloning to create a child provides some hope that our species is not inherently doomed. Bioethics alone is too weak a reed on which to build an international movement: human rights language is more powerful and has wider applicability. This is because it is not only medical and scientific practice that is at stake, but the nature of humanity and the rights of humans. Of course, because physician–researchers will pioneer all relevant experiments, bioethics remains pivotal even if not determinative. Let me conclude this chapter with a few modest suggestions.

On the national level, I have previously called for a moratorium on gene transfer experiments. That didn't happen, but the worldwide reassessment of gene transfer experiments makes such a moratorium less necessary. Nonetheless, we still need to ensure that all human gene transfer experiments, what are more commonly (and incorrectly) referred to as "gene therapy," be performed with full public knowledge and transparency.[44] A national debate on the goals of the research, and whether the lines between somatic cell and germline research, or between treatment and enhancement research, are meaningful should continue with more public involvement.[45] My own view is that the boundary line that really matters is set by the species itself and that species-endangering experiments should be outlawed.

We can take some actions on a national level, but we also need international rules about the new science, including not only cloning and genetic engineering (which will be discussed in more detail in the next chapter), but also human–machine cyborgs, xenografts, and brain alterations.[46] These could all fit into a *new category* of "crimes against humanity" in the strict sense, actions that threaten the integrity of the human species itself. This is not to say that changing the nature of humanity is always criminal, only that no individual scientist (or corporation or country) has the social or moral warrant to endanger humanity, including altering humans in ways that might endanger the species. Performing species-endangering experiments in the absence of social warrant, democratically developed, can properly be considered a terrorist act. Xenografts, for example, carry the risk of releasing a new, lethal virus upon humanity. No individual scientist or corporation has the moral warrant to risk this. Altering the human species in a way that predictably endangers it should require a worldwide discussion and debate, followed by a vote in an institution representative of the world's population, the United Nations being the only such entity today. It should also require a deep and wide-ranging discussion of our future and what kind of people we want to be, what kind of world we want to live in, and how we can protect universal human rights based on human dignity and democratic principles.

An international treaty banning specific species-endangering activities is necessary to make such a system effective. This, of course, begs two questions. First, exactly what types of human experiments should be prohibited? Second, what precisely is the international regime proposed? As to the first, the general definition could encompass all experimental interventions aimed at altering a fundamental characteristic of being human. There are at least two ways to change such characteristics. The first is to make a human trait optional. Changing it in one member (who continues to be seen as a member of the species) would change the species definition for everyone. An example is asexual replication cloning. When one human successfully engages in replication cloning, sexual reproduction will no longer be a necessary characteristic of being human. All humans will be capable of asexual replication. This will matter to all humans because it is not just our brains and what we can do with them (such as develop language and anticipate our deaths) that make us human, but also the interaction of our brains with our bodies.

A second way to change a characteristic of being human would be any alteration that would make the resulting person someone we *Homo sapiens* would no longer identify as a member of our species or who could not sexually reproduce with a human. Examples would include the insertion of an artificial chromosome that would make sexual reproduction impossible, as well as physically altering basic brain and body structure (for example, number of arms, legs, eyes, etc., and, of course, the addition of new appendages such as wings or new functional organs such as gills). This is important because the resulting person would likely be viewed as a new species or subspecies of humans, and thus not necessarily a possessor of all human rights.

Genetic engineering experiments not aimed at changing the nature of the species or at placing the resultant person outside the definition of *Homo sapiens* (such as those aimed at improving memory, immunity, strength, and other characteristics that some existing humans have) should also be subject to international oversight. Moreover, I don't think any of them should be performed on children, fetuses, or embryos. This is because of their inherent physical and psychological danger to children (and the overall danger they pose to children of treating them as manufactured products), and because there are existing alternative, less dangerous educational, exercise-based, medical, and surgical ways to achieve these goals. Parents should simply not be able to dominate their children in this fashion: what can be considered liberty for an adult is tyranny when forced on the next generation. Not included would be somatic cell interventions aimed at curing or preventing disease, although I believe these should be regulated on a national basis. An intermediate case might be the addition of an artificial gene to an embryo that could not be activated until adulthood—and then only by the individual. Proving such an intervention safe may, however, be an insurmountable problem.

To be effective, a "human species protection" treaty would have to describe and authorize an oversight and enforcement mechanism. The body to enforce the treaty should be an international administrative agency with rule-making and adjudicatory authority. The rule-making process would develop and promulgate the basic rules for species-endangering experiments. Adjudicatory authority would be necessary to determine if and when applications by researchers to perform the potentially species-endangering experiments would be approved, and to determine if individuals had violated the terms of the treaty. The agency I envision would not have criminal jurisdiction but could refer cases to the International Criminal Court.

As the next chapter elucidates, drafting and enacting such a treaty, even beginning the process, is a nontrivial undertaking and will require a sustained effort. In the meantime, individual governments, corporations, and professional associations can declare potentially species-endangering experiments off-limits. Such action would take human rights and democratic principles seriously and recognize that a risk to the entire species is one only the species itself can agree to take. To be effective, the treaty itself must provide that no species-endangering techniques be used unless and until the international body approved its use in humans. This would change the burden of proof and put it on the would-be species-endangerers. It would thus apply the environmental movement's precautionary principle to species-endangering experimentation.[47] That there is no such treaty and no such mechanism in place today signifies that the world community has not yet taken responsibility for its future. It is past time that we did. James Watson had it wrong. The truth is that at the beginning of the last millennium we *knew* that our future was in the stars; now, at the beginning of this millennium, we *think* that our future is in our genes.

We have a tendency simply to let science take us where it will. But science has no will, and human judgment is almost always necessary for any successful exploration of the unknown. Columbus's ships would have turned back but for his human courage and determination. And the first moon landing was almost a disaster because the computer overshot the planned landing site by four miles. Only the expert human piloting of Neil Armstrong was able to avert disaster. The first words from humans on the moon were not Armstrong's "one small step for man," but Buzz Aldrin's "Contact light! Okay, engine stop . . . descent engine command override off."[48] It is time for us humans to take command of spaceship Earth and turn on science's engine override command. This should greatly increase the likelihood that our species will survive in good health to experience another millennium.

4

. . . .

The Endangered Human

We humans tend to worry first about ourselves, then about our families, then about our communities. In times of great stress, such as war or natural disaster, we may focus temporarily on our country, but we almost never think about our planet as a whole or our species as a whole. This constricted perspective, perhaps best exemplified by the American consumer, has led to the environmental degradation of Earth, a gross and widening gap in living standards between rich and poor nations and people, and a scientific research agenda that focuses almost exclusively on the needs and desires of the wealthy West. Reversing worldwide trends toward market-based atomization and increasing indifference to the suffering of others will require a human rights focus forged by the development of what Vaclav Havel has termed a "species consciousness."

In this chapter I explore the blurring of boundaries between bioethics and human rights by discussing human cloning and inheritable genetic alterations from the human species perspective. In this context I also suggest language for a proposed international "Convention on the Preservation of the Human Species" that would outlaw all efforts to initiate a pregnancy using either intentionally modified genetic material or human replication cloning, such as through somatic cell nuclear transfer.[1] I sum-marize international legal action in these areas, relate these actions to argu-ments for and against a treaty, and conclude with an action plan.

Human Rights and the Human Species

The deployment of the atomic bomb not only presented the world for the first time with the prospect of total annihilation, but also, paradoxically, led to a renewed emphasis on the "nuclear family," complete with its per-sonal bomb shelter. The conclusion of World War II (with the dropping of the only two atomic bombs ever used in war) led to the recognition that world wars were now suicidal to the entire species and to the formation of the United Nations with the primary goal of preventing such wars. That we are all fundamentally the same, all human, with the same dignity and rights, is at the core of the United Nations Charter and the Universal Declaration of Human Rights.

Membership in the human species is central to the meaning and en-forcement of human rights, and respect for basic human rights is essential for the survival of the human species. The development of the concept of "crimes against humanity" was a milestone for universalizing human rights in that it recognized that there were certain actions, such as slavery and genocide, that implicated the entire species and so merited universal con-demnation.[2] Nuclear weapons were immediately recognized as a technology that requires international control, and so have extreme genetic manipula-tions such as cloning and inheritable genetic alterations. Both belong in the general category of species-endangering activities. In fact, cloning and inheritable genetic alterations can be seen as crimes against humanity of a unique sort: techniques that can alter the essence of humanity itself (and thus threaten to change the foundation of human rights as well) by taking human evolution into our own hands and directing it toward the develop-ment of a new species, sometimes termed the posthuman.[3] It may be that extreme species-altering techniques such as cloning and inheritable genetic modifications could provide benefits to the human species in extraordi-nary circumstances. For example, asexual replication could potentially save humans from extinction if all humans were rendered sterile by some cata-strophic event, transforming an otherwise species-endangering activity into a species-saving one.

As a baseline, if we take human rights and democracy seriously, a de-cision to alter a fundamental characteristic of humans should not be taken by any individual or corporation without wide discussion among all members of the affected population. As I concluded in the previous chapter, no individual scientist or corporation has the moral warrant to redesign humans (any more than any individual scientist or corporation has the moral warrant to design a new, lethal virus or bacteria that could kill large numbers of humans). Species-endangering experiments directly concern all humans and should only be authorized democratically by a body that is representative of everyone on the planet. These are the most important decisions we will ever make. The widespread condemnation of human replicative cloning by governments around the world provides a perhaps unique opportunity for the world to begin to work together to take some control over biotechnology that threatens our very existence.

The environmental movement has adopted the precautionary principle to help stem the tide of environmental alterations that are detrimental to humans. One version of this principle holds that "when an activity raises threats of harm to human health or the environment . . . the proponent of that activity, rather than the public, should bear the burden of proof [that the activity is more likely to be beneficial than harmful]."[4] The most effective way to shift the burden of proof is to outlaw dangerous and potentially lethal activities, thus requiring the proponents engaging in them to change the law before proceeding. This can be done nation-by-nation, but can only be made effective (because scientists and laboratories can move from country to country) by an internationally enforceable ban. The actual text of a treaty banning human replicative cloning and inheritable modifications is and will continue to be the subject of international debate. Following a national conference, Beyond Cloning, held at Boston University in September 2001 (two weeeks after 9/11), Lori Andrews and I suggested the following language (obviously subject to negotiation and added details) as a basis for going forward.[5]

Convention on the Preservation of the Human Species

The Parties to this Convention,

Noting that the Charter of the United Nations affirms human rights, based on the dignity and worth of the human person and on equal rights of all persons,

Noting that the Universal Declaration of Human Rights affirms the principle of the inadmissibility of discrimination,

Realizing that human dignity and human rights derive from our common humanity,

Noting the increased power of genetic science, which opens up vast prospects for improving health, but also has the power to fundamentally diminish humanity by producing a child through human cloning or through intentionally producing an inheritable genetic change,

Concerned that human cloning, which for the first time would produce children with predetermined genotypes, rather than novel genotypes, might cause these children to be deprived of their human rights,

Concerned that by altering fundamental human characteristics even to the extent of possibly producing a new human species or subspecies, genetic science will cause the resulting persons to be treated unequally or deprived of their human rights,

Recognizing the history of abuses of human rights in the name of genetic science,

Believing that no individual, nation, or corporation has the moral or legal warrant to engage in species-endangering procedures, including cloning and genetic alteration of reproductive cells or embryos for the creation of a child,

Believing that the creation of a new species or subspecies of humans could easily lead to genocide or slavery,

Stressing the need for global cooperation to prevent the misuse of genetic science in ways that undermine human dignity and human rights,

Have agreed on the following:

Article 1

Parties shall take all reasonable action, including the adoption of criminal laws, to prohibit anyone from initiating or attempting to initiate a human pregnancy or other form of gestation using embryos or reproductive cells which have undergone intentional inheritable genetic modification.

Article 2

Parties shall take all reasonable action, including the adoption of criminal laws, to prohibit anyone from utilizing somatic cell nuclear transfer or any other cloning technique for the purpose of initiating or attempting to initiate a human pregnancy or other form of gestation.

Article 3

Parties shall implement a system of national oversight through legislation, executive order, decree, or other mechanism to regulate facilities engaged in assisted human reproduction or otherwise using human gametes or embryos for experimentation or clinical purposes to ensure that such facilities meet informed consent, safety, and ethical standards.

Article 4

A Conference of the Parties and a Secretariat shall be established to oversee implementation of the Convention.

Article 5

Reservations to this Convention are not permitted.

Article 6

For the purpose of this Convention, the term "somatic cell nuclear transfer" shall mean transferring the nucleus of a human somatic cell into an ovum or oocyte. "Somatic cell" shall mean any cell of a human embryo, fetus, child or adult other than a reproductive cell. "Embryo" shall include a fertilized egg, zygote (including a blastomere and blastocyst), and preembryo. "Reproductive cell" shall mean a human gamete and its precursors.

Perhaps the most difficult challenge in implementing this treaty would be setting up the monitoring and enforcement mechanisms. The Article 4 process would have to address these. In general terms, monitoring and compliance bodies would have to be broadly representative, possess authority to oversee activities related to cloning and human genetic modification, and be able to enforce bans by announcing and denouncing potential violators. It also seems reasonable to support two new international crimes: initiation of a pregnancy to create a human clone, and initiation of a pregnancy using a genetically altered embryo.

Why an International Convention?

More than seven years after the announcement of the cloning of Dolly the sheep, it is time to ask not if cloning and germ line genetic alterations should be regulated, but how. Had a five-year moratorium for further thought and discussion been placed on cloning humans, as the National Bioethics Advisory Commission recommended in 1997, for example, the time would long since have expired.[6] What have we learned since Dolly's birth?

First, virtually every scientist in the world with an opinion believes it is unsafe to attempt a human pregnancy with a cloned embryo. This was, for example, the unanimous conclusion of a 2002 report from the U.S. National Academy of Sciences, which recommended that human "reproductive" cloning be outlawed in the United States.[7] Although scientists seldom like to predict the future without overwhelming data to support them, many believe human cloning or inheritable genetic alternations at the embryo level will never be safe because they will always be inherently unpredictable in their effects on the children and their offspring. As embryologist Stewart Newman has noted, for example, it is unlikely that a human created from the union of "two damaged cells" (an enucleated egg and a nucleus removed from a somatic cell) could ever be healthy.[8] Of course, adding genetic modification to the somatic cell's nucleus adds another series of events that could go wrong, because genes seldom have a single function but interact in complex and unpredictable ways with other genes.[9] It is worth emphasizing that the dangers are not only physical, but also psychological. Whether cloned children could ever overcome the psychological problems associated with their origins is unknown and perhaps unknowable.[10] In short, the safety issues, which make attempts to clone or genetically alter a human being inherently unethical human experiments, provide sufficient scientific justification for the treaty.

If and when safety can be assured, assuming this will ever be possible, two primary arguments have been put forth in favor of proceeding with cloning (and its first cousin, inheritable genetic alterations): cloning is a type of human reproduction that can help infertile couples have genetically related children, and cloning is a part of human progress (that could lead to a new type of genetic immortality), so that to prevent it is to be antiscientific.

The infertility argument is made by physiologist Panos Zavos and his former colleague, Italian infertility specialist Severino Antinori. They argue that the inability of a sterile male to have a genetically related child is such a human tragedy that it justifies human cloning.[11] This view not only ignores the rights and interests of women and children (even if only males are to be cloned, eggs must be procured from a woman, the embryos gestated by a woman, and the child is the subject of the experiment), but also contains a highly contested assertion: that asexual genetic replication or duplication should be seen as human reproduction.[12] In fact humans are a sexually reproducing species and have never reproduced or replicated themselves asexually.

Asexual replication may or may not be categorized by future courts as a form of human reproduction, but there are strong arguments against it. First, the option of asexual reproduction displaces a fundamental characteristic of what it means to be human (a sexually reproducing species) by making sexual reproduction involving the genetic mixture of male and female gametes optional. Second, the "child" in asexual replication is also the twin of the genetic parent, a relationship that has never existed in human society. The first clone, for example, will be the first human being with a single genetic parent (unless his biological grandparents are taken to be the actual parents of the clone). Third, the genetic replica of a genetically sterile man is himself sterile and can "reproduce" only by cloning. This means either that infertility is not a major problem (because if it were, it would be unethical for a physician to intentionally create a child with this problem), or that the desire of existing adults should take precedence over the welfare of children. Neither conclusion is persuasive, and this is probably why, although some ethicists believe that cloning could be considered a form of human reproduction, infertility specialists have not joined Zavos and Antinori's call for human cloning as a treatment for infertile males. In fact, the organization that represents infertility specialists in the United States and that is generally opposed to the regulation of infertility treatment, the American Society of Reproductive Medicine, has consistently opposed human cloning.[13]

There are, nonetheless, legal commentators who believe that human cloning should be classified as a form of human reproduction, and constitutionally protected as such, at least if it is the only way for an individual to have a "genetically related child." The strongest proponent of this view is probably John Robertson,[14] although Ronald Dworkin[15] shares his enthusiasm. Suffice it to respond that it is very unclear that human reproduction or procreation of a kind protected by principles of autonomy and self-fulfillment can be found in a "right to have a genetically related child." As Leon Kass, the head of the President's Council on Bioethics, has noted in another context, it cannot be just the genetic tie that is important in human reproduction, because if it were, this could be accomplished by having one's identical twin brother have a child with one's wife[16]—the genetic tie would be identical, yet few, if any, would argue that this method of reproduction would satisfy the twin's right to have a "genetically related child." Moreover, in cloning, the *genetic* relationship is not a parent–child relationship at all, but a sibling relationship. Genes are important, but there is more to human reproduction, as protected by the U.S. Constitution, than simple genetic replication.

The second major argument in favor of human cloning is that it can produce a form of immortality. This is the premise of the Raelian cult, which has formed its own corporation, Clonaid, to engage in human cloning. The leader of the cult, who calls himself Rael (formerly Claude Vorilhon, the editor of a French motor sports magazine), believes that all humans were created in the laboratories of the planet Elohim and that the Elohims have instructed Rael and his followers to develop cloning on Earth to provide earthlings with a form of immortality.[17] The Raelians, of course, can believe whatever they want, but just as human sacrifices are outlawed, so too can be experiments that pose a significant danger to women and children, and the religious beliefs of this cult do not provide a sufficient justification to refrain from outlawing cloning.

Two basic arguments about the future regulation of these technologies have also emerged. The first, enunciated by Lee Silver, is that these technologies, while not necessarily desirable, are unstoppable because the market combined with parental desire will drive scientists and physicians to offer these services to demanding couples. As parents now seek early educational enrichment for their children, parents of the future will seek early genetic enhancement to give their children a competitive advantage in life. Silver believes this will ultimately lead to the creation of two separate species or subspecies, the "GenRich" and "the naturals."[18]

A related "do nothing" argument is that regulation may not be needed because the technologies will not be widely used. The thought is that humans may muddle through either because the science of human genetic alterations may never prove possible, or because it will be used by only a handful of humans because most will instinctively reject it. Steven Pinker is probably the most articulate spokesperson for this view. He argues that at least as long as genetic engineering of children remains a risky business, few parents will actually be willing to risk the health of their future children for a speculative genetic improvement.[19] Pinker may be correct, but he may not be. In any event, his arguments do not negate the desirability of a democratically formed regulatory scheme.[20]

The primary arguments against cloning and inheritable genetic alterations are that these interventions would require massive dangerous and unethical human experimentation,[21] that cloning would inevitably be harmful to the resulting children by restricting their liberty,[22] that cloning would lead to a new eugenics movement for "designer children" (because if an individual could pick the entire genome of their future child, it would seem impossible to prohibit individuals from picking one or more specific genetic characteristics of their future children),[23] and that it would likely lead to the creation of a new species or subspecies of humans, the posthuman.[24] In the context of the species, the last argument has gotten the least attention, and so it is worth saying more about what the creation of a posthuman would mean.

The core argument is that cloning will inevitably lead us down a slippery slope to attempts to modify the somatic cell nucleus to create not genetic duplicates of existing people, but "better" children.[25] This attempt will either succeed or fail. If it fails, that is the end of it. If it succeeds, however, something like the scenario envisioned by Silver and others, such as Nancy Kress, will unfold: a new species or subspecies of humans will emerge.[26] The new species, or posthumans, will likely view the old "normal" humans as inferiors, even savages, and fit for slavery or slaughter. The normals, on the other hand, may see the posthumans as a threat, and if they can, engage in a preemptive strike by killing the posthumans before they themselves are killed or enslaved by them.

It is the predictable potential for genocide, which I have termed "genetic genocide," that makes extreme species-altering experiments potential weapons of mass destruction and makes the unaccountable genetic engineer a potential bioterrorist. This is one reason why cloning and inheritable genetic modification is of specieswide concern and why an international treaty to address this category of species-endangering activity is needed. Such a treaty is necessary because existing laws on cloning and inheritable alterations, even though often well-intentioned, have serious limitations. Some are mere moratoria and have already expired. Some are limited in the type of species-altering technologies they ban, covering only cloning and not germline genetic interventions, or even just applying to cloning in a limited range of techniques. Some of the existing laws have also been outpaced by technology and do not apply to comprehensively ban all forms of replicative cloning and germline interventions. Others are ambiguous about what they cover. In some cases, potentially relevant laws were adopted more than two decades ago to deal with a different set of technologies and concerns; it is unclear whether their expansive prohibitions will be applied to the newer technologies of reproductive cloning and germline intervention. Moreover, many of the existing declarations and laws do not include appropriate sanctions. And, of course, scientists can engage in regulatory arbitrage by crossing national borders to do their research in a country without a prohibition.[27]

Numerous international entities have called for an enforceable ban on human cloning. The World Health Organization (WHO) at its 51st World Health Assembly reaffirmed that "cloning for replication of human beings is ethically unacceptable and contrary to human dignity and integrity." WHO urges member states to "foster continued and informed debate on these issues and to take appropriate steps, including legal and juridical measures, to prohibit cloning for the purpose of replicating human individuals." The European Union's Council of Europe adopted the Council of Europe Protocol, prohibiting the cloning of human beings. Similarly, the European Parliament has adopted a Resolution on Human Cloning. The resolution calls for member states to enact binding national legislation to ban cloning and also urges the United Nations to secure an international ban on cloning. Likewise, UNESCO's Universal Declaration on the Human Genome and Human Rights specifically addresses cloning and states "Practices which are contrary to human dignity, such as reproductive cloning of human beings, shall not be permitted."

The Treaty Process

On August 7, 2001, France and Germany urged the United Nations Secretary-General to add to the UN's agenda an international convention against reproductive cloning of human beings. In November 2001 the Legal Committee of the UN added its support and held meetings in 2002 and 2003.

No country wants to allow use of the "Dolly the sheep" cloning technique—the one since used to create mice, pigs, cows, and, most recently, rabbits and kittens—to make a human child. Virtually every nation agrees that children should not be commodified like barnyard animals or pets, even like beloved cats and dogs. The powerful global consensus that human reproductive cloning should be outlawed provides an unprecedented opportunity for the world to take united action on a bioethical issue that could profoundly affect the future of our species.

The United States, nonetheless, threatened to take its ball and go home if the world community did not give in to its demands to outlaw not just reproductive cloning but also research cloning. (Sometimes called "therapeutic cloning"—though no therapies have been produced—research cloning involves making human embryos by somatic cell nuclear transfer with the goal of deriving stem cells for medical research.) This all-or-nothing, take-it-or-leave-it approach is the same position taken by the House of Representatives and repeated by President George W. Bush (although not by his Council on Bioethics). With treaty cosponsors France and Germany also opposing the war with Iraq, the U.S. government was perhaps even less disposed than usual to take bioethics lessons from these countries.

To date, the U.S. Senate has never even debated the ban, probably because the outcome remains too close to call. Nonetheless, unless a compromise can ultimately be reached so that outlawing reproductive cloning is not held hostage to banning research cloning, the likely outcome is that no law will ever pass. Without congressional action to ban reproductive cloning in the United States, it will probably be attempted by its radical proponents. Is there a compromise that can stop the cloning renegades while permitting legitimate medical research?

The first step toward a solution is to understand the Bush administration's position. Leon Kass, its intellectual architect, has argued eloquently and passionately that if you oppose creating a child by cloning, you must also oppose creating human embryos for research by cloning. This is because, he says, if research cloning is permitted, it is inevitable that someone will try to implant one of the cloned embryos in a woman, and once this occurs, no government would ever force the woman to abort the clone. Moreover, he argues, research cloning would result in private industry stockpiling human embryos and mining, exploiting, and selling them. Opponents of research cloning have run radio ads warning of "embryo hatcheries" and "embryo farms." A ban on implanting these embryos, Kass says, would require the government to destroy cloned embryos rather than preserve and protect this form of nascent human life, action that would be repugnant to many.

Kass reiterated this position in 2002, when he opened the first meeting of the Presidents' Council on Bioethics with a discussion of Nathaniel Hawthorne's "The Birthmark." In the story, a scientist, Aylmer, marries a beautiful young woman, Georgiana, who has a small handlike birthmark on her face. Aylmer becomes obsessed with removing it, and the potion he ultimately creates to successfully remove it also kills her. Imperfection, of course, is an inherent characteristic of humans, and attempting to make the perfect human is certainly dangerous and ultimately impossible. Kass takes the story as a cautionary tale that science's attempt to perfect humans by, among other things, changing our basic sexual nature (by making sexual reproduction optional) could have deadly consequences.

Kass (and Bush, and the United States with its anti–research cloning allies at the United Nations) is right to caution us about the limits of our technology and the slippery slope. Aylmer was wrong to see human perfection through scientific technique as a reasonable human goal, and "The Birthmark" rightly warns us about that nightmarish eugenic goal. But is the United States right to oppose research cloning aimed at finding cures for devastating human diseases and alleviating severe human suffering, historically both important and completely legitimate goals of medical research? I don't think so, at least not if we can take effective regulatory steps. And this points the way to a possible political compromise.

There are two basic ways the Senate could act to stop baby-making cloners without outlawing research on cloned embryos. The first, as suggested by the Bioethics Council in July 2002, is to put a moratorium on research cloning until the use of adult stem cells is fully explored and/or until research using stem cells from "spare," or leftover, embryos created at in vitro fertilization clinics is demonstrated to be of therapeutic value in tissue regeneration. The second and, I think, better and more permanent solution is to create a regulatory regime that would make the administration's dreaded commercial stockpiles (and farms) of cloned embryos and the initiation of a pregnancy with one of them virtually impossible.

Regulation would be a challenge. Historically, embryo research has never been federally regulated, primarily because the U.S. government has never funded it. Nonetheless, Congress has the authority to regulate all such research, not just publicly funded research, if it wants to. In particular, Congress could greatly improve the overall ethics of now unregulated research with cloned human embryos, permitting the science to proceed, and at the same time virtually guarantee that no cloned human embryo lawfully made would be implanted—or have to be ordered destroyed by the government. Here is how it would work. Ideally, Congress would create a federal oversight authority (similar to England's Human Fertilization and Embryology Authority) that would have exclusive authority to permit any proposed embryo research project, including those in the private sector. Approval would only be granted for those projects soundly designed to address a compelling medical need that could be successfully addressed no other way.

To prevent the transgressions envisioned by Kass and the Bush administration, specifically the stockpiling and commercial use of cloned research embryos and the implanting of a research embryo to start a pregnancy, at least three prohibitions would be required. The freezing and storage of cloned embryos would be outlawed. Cloned embryos would be created solely for use in approved research projects, and there would be no reason to "store" or "stockpile" them because the research embryos would be destroyed in the research process. A strict limit of seven days would be placed on the length of time any cloned human embryo could be maintained. The purchase and sale of human eggs and human embryos would be outlawed. This would help to eliminate the increasing commercialization of embryo research and the commodification of both human eggs and embryos. All individuals, including physicians, scientists, and biotech companies not approved to do research cloning, would be prohibited from making or possessing cloned embryos. In addition, all in vitro fertilization clinics and physicians and embryologists associated with them would be specifically prohibited from doing research on cloned embryos—making it virtually impossible for a cloned embryo ever to be used to initiate a pregnancy.[28]

Aylmer's real crime was that he was unable to separate his love for his wife from his love of science, and in joining them he killed her. Combining bans on both reproductive and research cloning in one bill is likely to kill the anticloning legislation as well. And because reasonable compromise is available, this lethal outcome is unnecessary. We can sketch a parallel from another regulatory realm that helps demonstrate that the law can effectively ban one activity without banning two related activities. There is a reasonable argument that an effective ban on offensive biological weapons research requires a ban on defensive biological weapons research as well. Nonetheless, it would be self-defeating and irrational to refuse to support a ban on offensive weapons research solely because defensive research was not banned simultaneously. Defensive biowarfare research can be used to make an offensive weapon, of course, but this requires both a greater volume of toxins as well as a delivery system. Likewise, cloned embryos could be used to make babies, but we are much more likely to prevent this eventuality with a ban on implanting cloned human embryos coupled with regulation of embryo research than with no regulation of cloning at all. We can outlaw cloning to create children without outlawing cloning to create medicines.

Actions of the U.S. Senate and the United States at the United Nations are a moving target. Nonetheless, as of this writing the United States has managed to persuade almost 80 other countries to support its position that no treaty prohibiting reproductive cloning should be adopted that does not also outlaw research cloning, and the treaty drafting process has stalled. Until this impasse is broken, it seems likely that no federal law will be enacted in the United States, and without strong U.S. support and leadership, no cloning treaty will be adopted at the United Nations. One possible compromise is to put cloning to one side for now and concentrate exclusively on the real species-endangering activity, inheritable genetic alteration, since there is currently no support for this activity by any government or scientific organization in the world.

Conclusion

Biotechnology, especially human cloning and germline genetic engineering, has the potential to permit us to design our children and to literally change the characteristics of the human species. The movement toward a posthuman world can be characterized as progress and enhancement of individual freedom in the area of procreation, but it also can be characterized as a movement down a slippery slope to a neoeugenics that will result in the creation of one or more subspecies or superspecies of humans. The first vision sees science as our guide and ultimate goal. The second is more firmly based on evidence from our history, which has consistently identified differences and has used those differences to justify genocidal actions. It is the prospect of "genetic genocide" that calls for treating cloning and genetic engineering as potential weapons of mass destruction and the unaccountable genetic researcher as a potential bioterrorist.

The greatest accomplishment of humans has not been our science, but our development of human rights and democracy. Science deals with facts, not values. Since science cannot tell us what we should do, or even what our goals are, humans must give direction to science. In the area of genetics, this calls for international action to oversee the techniques that could lead us to commit species suicide. We humans recognized the risk in splitting the atom and developing nuclear weapons, and most humans recognize the risk in using human genes to modify ourselves. Since the risk is to the entire species, it requires a species response. Many countries have already enacted bans, moratoria, and strict regulations on various species-altering technologies. The challenge, however, is global, and action on the international level is required for oversight to be effective.

One action called for is the ratification of an international convention for the preservation of the human species that outlaws human replication cloning and inheritable alterations. This ban would not only be important in and of itself, it would also mark the first time the world worked together to limit a biotechnology. Cloning and germline genetic modifications are not bioweapons per se, but they could prove just as destructive to the human species if left to the market and individual wants and desires. An international consensus to ban these technologies for reproductive use already exists, and countries, nongovernmental organizations, and individual citizens should actively support the treaty process, as they did with the Convention on the Prohibition of the Use, Stockpiling, Production and Transfer of Anti-Personnel Mines and their Destruction (Mine Ban Treaty).

Cloning may not seem as important as land mines because no clone has yet been born and thus no children have yet been harmed by this technique or by using it to produce inheritable alterations. Nonetheless, cloning has the potential to harm all children, both directly by limiting the clones' freedom and harming them physically and mentally and indirectly by devaluing all children through treating them as products of their parents' genetic specifications. Of more concern, inheritable genetic alteration carries the prospect of developing a new species of humans who could turn into either destroyers or victims of the human species. Opposition to cloning and inheritable genetic alteration is conservative in the strict sense of the word: it seeks to conserve the human species. But it is also liberal in the strict sense of the word: it seeks to preserve democracy, freedom, and universal human rights for all members of the human species.

Proponents of going full speed ahead with inheritable genetic alterations are fond of quoting Thucydides's *History of the Peloponnesian War* to the effect that, "The bravest are surely those with the clearest vision of the future, disaster and benefit alike, and that not withstanding these possibilities they move ahead." It sounds great, but when placed in historical context, the statement actually supports application of the precautionary principle to inheritable genetic alterations. The statement is made by the revered Athenian general Pericles in his famous funeral oration praising the nature of Athenian citizenship. His real point is not that Athenians are impulsive and brave, but rather that as a democracy they think before they act and weigh the possible consequences before voting on how to proceed. As Pericles puts it concisely, "the worst thing is to rush into action before the consequences have been properly debated."[29] And later, when Athens is in the midst of a disastrous war, Thucydides, a former general himself, describes how war changes what we think of as virtue:

> What used to be described as a thoughtless act of aggression was now regarded as courage ... to think of the future and wait was merely another way of saying one was a coward ... ability to understand a question from all sides meant that one was totally unfitted for action. Fanatical enthusiasm was the mark of a real man.[30]

This chapter has dealt with trying to avoid technologically induced catastrophies that would necessitate a funeral oration by a posthuman Pericles stand-in on behalf of the human species itself. In the next chapter I take up a more immediate topic, the right to health.

5

. . . .

The Right to Health

Activists in South Africa succeeded in returning health as a human right to the international stage just as it was being displaced by economists who see health through the prism of a globalized economy and politicians who see it as an issue of national security or charity.[1] The current postapartheid debate in South Africa is not about race, but about health, and in this context the court victory by AIDS activists regarding nevirapine has been termed not only "the greatest defeat for Mbeki's government" but also the opening of "legitimate criticism" of the government "over a host of issues from land rights to the pursuit of wealth."[2] Using the South African nevirapine case as a centerpiece, in this chapter I explore the utility of the often misunderstood international human right to health to improve health generally.

Jonathan Mann rightly observed that "health and human rights are inextricably linked,"[3] and Paul Farmer has argued that "the most important question facing modern medicine involves human rights." Farmer noted that many poor people have no access to modern medicine, concluding, "The more effective the treatment, the greater the injustice meted out to those who do not have access to care."[4] Access to treatment for HIV/AIDS has been problematic in almost every country but has perhaps been most frustrating in South Africa, where more than 5 million people are infected with HIV and the government's attitude toward the HIV/AIDS epidemic has been described as pseudoscientific and dangerous.[5] Political resistance by the South African government to outside funders who seek to set the country's health care agenda is, of course, understandable in the context of a history of racism and colonialism.[6] But understandable politics cannot excuse the government's failure to act decisively in the face of an unprecedented epidemic.

HIV Infection and the Right to Health

One of the most controversial actions of the South African government has been its drastic restriction of the use of nevirapine to prevent the transmission of HIV from mother to infant. The Treatment Action Campaign, a coalition of South African AIDS-related organizations, was formed in 1998 to promote affordable treatment to all people with HIV infection or AIDS. This group (and others) celebrated a victory in 2001 when 39 multinational pharmaceutical companies withdrew their lawsuit against the South African government to enforce patents on HIV/AIDS treatment drugs, which would have prevented the government from purchasing generic versions.[7] At about the same time, the Treatment Action Campaign itself brought suit against the South African government. The suit alleged that governmental restrictions on the availability of nevirapine (limiting it in the public sector to hospitals involved in a pilot study) and the failure to have a reasonable government plan to make the drug more widely available violated the right to health of South African HIV-positive pregnant women and their children. The use of nevirapine remains controversial in Africa, even after a Uganda study published in 1999 suggested that administering the drug to a pregnant woman at the outset of labor and to her newborn immediately after birth could result in a 50 percent reduction in the rate of transmission of HIV.[8] This study was the basis for the claim that failure to use nevirapine condemns 35,000 newborns a year to HIV infection in South Africa.

The Treatment Action Campaign prevailed in the trial court, which ruled that restricting nevirapine to a limited number of pilot sites in the public sector "is not reasonable and is an unjustifiable barrier to the progressive realization of the right to health care."[9] In July 2002, in *Treatment Action Campaign v. Minister of Health*, the Constitutional Court of South Africa, the country's highest court, affirmed, ruling that the government's nevirapine policy violated the health care rights of women and newborns under the South African constitution.[10] The postapartheid constitution provides in relevant part:

Section 27. Health care, food, water, and social security

(1) Everyone has the right to have access to
    (a) health care services, including reproductive health care;
    (b) sufficient food and water; and
    (c) social security . . .
(2) The state must take reasonable legislative and other measures, within its available resources, to achieve the progressive realization of each of these rights.
(3) No one may be refused emergency medical treatment.

Section 28. Children

(1) Every child has a right . . .
    (b) to family care or parental care, or to appropriate alternative care when removed from the family environment;
    (c) to basic nutrition, shelter, basic health care services and social services; . . .
(2) A child's best interests are of paramount importance in every matter concerning the child . . .

These rights are part of the bill of rights in the South African constitution, which the constitution itself requires the state to "respect, protect, promote and fulfill." These provisions are modeled on those in the International Covenant on Economic, Social, and Cultural Rights (which has been signed but not yet ratified by South Africa). Under the covenant (reprinted in Appendix C) the right to health in Article 12 includes not only appropriate health care but also a right to the underlying determinants of health, including clean water, adequate sanitation, safe food, housing, and health-related education. South Africa's constitutional health obligations apply to every branch of government. The Constitutional Court considered two questions: what actions the government was required to take with regard to nevirapine, and whether the government had an obligation to establish a comprehensive plan for the prevention of HIV transmission from mother to child.

Making Nevirapine Available

As justification for its refusal to make nevirapine available in public clinics, the South African government argued that the drug's safety and efficacy had not been satisfactorily determined and that it was of limited benefit in a breast-feeding population (since the number of infants acquiring HIV from breast feeding would be as large as the number infected without nevirapine use). These views were articulated by the minister of health, who, along with President Mbeki, has taken positions on HIV/AIDS and its treatment that scientists in the rest of the world find simply baffling.

In January 2001, after a meeting of southern African countries, the World Health Organization recommended the administration of nevirapine to HIV-positive mothers and their children at the time of birth. In April 2001 the Medicines Control Council, South Africa's equivalent of the Food and Drug Administration, formally approved nevirapine as safe and effective. Shortly thereafter, in July 2001, the government decided to conduct the pilot study of nevirapine at issue in the lawsuit. The study limited nevirapine's availability to two sites in each province. The result was that physicians who worked in the public sector at other facilities were unable to prescribe nevirapine for their patients, even though the manufacturer of the drug, Boehringer Ingelheim, had agreed to make it available at no cost for a five-year period. The Treatment Action Campaign argued that in the face of the HIV epidemic, which includes the infection of approximately 70,000 infants from their mothers annually, it was irrational and a breach of the bill of rights for the government to prohibit physicians in public clinics from prescribing nevirapine for preventive purposes when medically indicated.

The Obligation to Respect Rights

The government has an obligation to respect, protect, promote, and fulfill the right to health. The obligation to respect the right to health is primarily negative, requiring the government to refrain from denying or limiting equal access for all persons. *Treatment Action Campaign* was the third case in which the Constitutional Court had been asked to enforce a socioeconomic right under the constitution. The first case, *Soobramoney*, was also a right-to-health case.[11] It involved the claim by a 41-year-old man who, following a stroke, heart disease, and diabetes, suffered chronic renal failure, and because he was not eligible for a kidney transplant, required lifelong dialysis to survive. The renal dialysis unit in the region where he lived had 20 dialysis machines, many too few to dialyze everyone. It therefore had a policy of accepting only patients suffering from acute renal failure. The health department argued that this policy met their duty to provide emergency care under the constitution. Chronic renal sufferers, like the petitioner, did not automatically qualify for dialysis. In considering whether the constitution required the health department to provide a sufficient number of machines to dialyze everyone whose life could be saved by dialysis, the court observed that under the constitution the state's obligation to provide health care services was qualified by its "available resources." The court also noted that making extremely expensive medical treatments available to everyone would make "substantial inroads into the health budget . . . to the prejudice of the other needs which the state has to meet."

The Constitutional Court in *Soobramoney* ultimately decided that provincial health services administrators were the ones who should set budget priorities. Courts should not interfere with decisions that are rational and "taken in good faith by the political organs and medical authorities whose responsibility it is to deal with such matters." Likewise, in *Grootboom*, a case involving the right to housing, the Constitutional Court determined that although the state was obligated to act positively to ameliorate the conditions of the homeless, "the state is not obligated to go beyond available resources or to realize these rights immediately." The constitutional requirement is that the right to housing be "progressively realized." Nonetheless, the court noted that there is "at the very least, a negative obligation placed upon the state and all other entities and persons to desist from preventing or impairing the right of access to adequate housing."[12]

Applying these two cases to the *Treatment Action Campaign* case, the Constitutional Court reasonably concluded that the right to health care services "does not give rise to a self-standing and independent fulfillment right" enforceable irrespective of available resources. Nonetheless, the obligation to respect rights articulated in the housing decision applies equally to the right to health care services.

The Obligation to Protect and Fulfill Rights

The obligation to protect the right to health involves duties of states to adopt legislation or take other actions to ensure equal access to health care provided by third parties. The obligation to fulfill the right to health requires the state to adopt a national health policy with a detailed plan to implement the right to health. The Constitutional Court reframed the two questions it would answer in light of the South African government's obligation to take "reasonable steps" for the "progressive realization" of the right to health as: "is the policy of confining the supply of nevirapine reasonable in the circumstances, and does the government have a comprehensive policy for the prevention of mother-to-child transmission of HIV?"

The South African government argued that the real cost of delivering nevirapine is not the cost of the drug but the cost of the infrastructure of care: HIV testing, counseling, follow-up, and the provision of feeding formula for those who cannot afford it. The Constitutional Court agreed that the prevention ideal is to have these services universally available but restated the dispute as follows: "whether it was reasonable to exclude the use of nevirapine for the treatment of mother-to-child transmission at those public hospitals and clinics where testing and counseling are available."

The South African government gave four reasons for restricting nevirapine use: its efficacy would be diminished in settings in which a comprehensive package of services, including breast milk substitutes, was not available; its administration might produce a drug-resistant form of HIV; the safety of nevirapine had not been adequately demonstrated; and the public health system did not have the current capacity to deliver the "full package" of services. The court addressed each issue in turn. As to efficacy, the court found that breastfeeding did increase the risk of HIV infections "in some, but not all cases and that nevirapine thus remains to some extent efficacious . . . even if the mother breastfeeds her baby." As to drug resistance, the court conceded this possibility, but concluded, "The prospects of the child surviving if infected are so slim and the nature of the suffering so grave that the risk of some resistance manifesting at some time in the future is well worth running." The safety issue was disposed of by reference to the World Health Organization's recommendation of nevirapine and the determination of the Medicines Control Council that the drug was safe. As for capacity, the court concluded that resources are relevant to universal delivery of the "full package" but are "not relevant to the question of whether nevirapine should be used to reduce mother-to-child transmission of HIV at those public hospitals and clinics outside the research sites where facilities in fact exist for testing and counseling."

The Rights of Children and the Obligation to Fulfill Rights

This case is a right to health case because it concerns the availability of a drug and the circumstances under which the government can reasonably restrict its use. Nonetheless, this case could also have been decided solely on the rights of children. In the words of the Constitutional Court, "This case is concerned with newborn babies whose lives might be saved by the administration of nevirapine to mother and child at the time of birth." The court specifically cited the constitutional rights of children, including their right to "basic health care services." Parents have the primary obligation to provide these services to children but often cannot meet this obligation without help from the state.[13] The court concluded that nevirapine is an "essential" drug for children whose mothers are infected with HIV, that the needs of these children are "most urgent," and that their ability to exercise all other rights is "most in peril." The court did not write about the certainty of the children becoming orphans if their mothers did not also have access to treatment, but treatment was beyond the scope of this HIV prevention case.

On the basis of either the right to health or the rights of children, the court's answer to the first question was that the policy of restricting nevirapine to research settings was unreasonable and a violation of the government's obligation to take "reasonable legislative and other measures, within its available resources, to achieve the progressive realization" of the right to "access to health care services, including reproductive health care." In the court's words: "A potentially lifesaving drug was on offer and where testing and counseling facilities were available it could have been administered within the available resources of the state without any known harm to mother and child." The question of whether the cost of nevirapine mattered was not addressed, although the case almost certainly would have been decided differently had nevirapine not been available at no or very low cost.

The answer to the second question—whether the government is required to have a reasonable, comprehensive plan to combat mother-to-child transmission of HIV—flowed directly from the answer to the first. The legal question was whether the government's plan of moving slowly from limited research and training programs to more available programs was reasonable. The court decided that because of the "incomprehensible calamity" of the HIV epidemic in South Africa the government's slow-moving plan was not reasonable.

The Right to Progressive Realization of Health

Can the Constitutional Court be accused of playing the role of the South African government's health department in deciding how money should be spent on health care? The court did not think so. All branches of the government have the obligation to "respect, protect, promote and fulfill" the socio-economic rights contained in the constitution. As noted earlier, part of the obligation to fulfill requires the legislative branch to pass "reasonable legislative" measures, and the executive branch is obligated to develop and implement "appropriate, well-directed policies and programs." It is, of course, the role of the judiciary to resolve actual disputes as to whether specific legislation, policy, or implementation is consistent with the terms of the constitution. After the initiation of the lawsuit, three of the country's nine provinces, Western Cape, Gauteng, and KwaZulu-Natal, publicly announced a plan to progressively realize "the rights of pregnant women and their newborn babies to have access to nevirapine." The court expected the other six provinces to follow suit.

The court was explicit both in defining the rights that were violated and in ordering a remedy. As to the rights, the court declared that "Sections 27(1) and (2) of the Constitution require the government to devise and implement within its available resources a comprehensive and coordinated program to realize progressively the rights of pregnant women and their newborn children to have access to health services to combat mother-to-child transmission of HIV." To implement this right the court ordered the government to take four specific actions:

- Remove the restrictions that prevent nevirapine from being made available . . . at public hospitals and clinics that are not research and training sites.
- Permit and facilitate the use of nevirapine . . . at public hospitals and clinics when . . . this is medically indicated . . .
- Make provision if necessary for counselors based at public hospitals and clinics . . . to be trained for counseling . . .
- Take reasonable measures to extend the testing and counseling facilities at hospitals and clinics throughout the public health sector to facilitate and expedite the use of nevirapine.

Implementing the Right to Health

The *Treatment Action Campaign* decision illustrates both the strength and the weakness of relying on courts to determine specific applications of the right to health. The strength is that the right to health is a legal right, and since there can be no legal right without a remedy, this means that courts will provide a remedy for violations of the right to health. In this regard, it is worth noting that not only has the right to health and access to health care articulated in the Universal Declaration of Human Rights been given more specific meaning by the International Covenant on Economic, Social, and Cultural Rights and other internationally binding documents on human rights, but also that these rights have been written into the constitutions of more than 60 countries, including South Africa. The widespread failure of governments to take the right to health seriously, however, means that we are still far from the realization of this right. Nonetheless, the recent activism of many new nongovernmental organizations in the health rights area, such as the Treatment Action Campaign, provides some ground for optimism that government inaction will not go unchallenged.[14]

The weakness of relying on courts is that the focus in a courtroom struggle is likely to be narrow, involving specific medical interventions such as chronic kidney dialysis or nevirapine. Should nevirapine not turn out to be the drug of choice, either because it causes resistance in the mothers or because it is less effective than other approaches, the opinion will not help HIV-positive patients to obtain care. This is because the court's ruling is based on the assumption that nevirapine is safe and effective. The HIV/AIDS epidemic demands a comprehensive treatment and prevention strategy, including education, adequate nutrition, clean water, and gender equality.[15] It will take even more, as South African physician and medical ethicist Solomon Benatar has concluded, because "improvement of health in South Africa will depend both on enlightened, vigorous reconsideration of many local policies and practices and on the reshaping of the global forces that affect the health of whole populations."[16]

Nelson Mandela has accurately noted that an effective national HIV/AIDS strategy requires the engaged commitment of national leaders to provide not only prevention but also treatment for everyone who needs it "wherever they may be in the world and regardless of whether they can afford to pay or not."[17] The market currently decides who lives and who dies. The ongoing WHO/UNAIDS "3 by 5" initiative, which aims to start three million patients on antiretroviral treatments by the end of 2005, "proposes that governments consider universal access to AIDS treatment to be a basic human right in accordance with the Universal Declaration of Human Rights, which recognizes the right to health care and the right to share in the advances of science."[18] This right to health philosophy merits the active support of bioethicists everywhere, especially in the world's richest country where health care has yet to be recognized as a right.

In the next chapter I move from economic and social rights to political and civil rights, with the extreme example of capital punishment and the physician's role as an agent of the state.

6

. . . .

Capital Punishment

Kant postulated that humans as a species move progressively to a more moral state. In his words, "since the human race's natural end is to make steady cultural progress, its moral end is to be conceived as progressing toward the better. And this progress may well be occasionally interrupted, but it will never be broken off."[1] Capital punishment provides a profitable case study in moral progress. Because capital punishment has been medicalized by adopting lethal injection as its methodology (sometimes termed "killing with kindness"), and because medicalization is critical to capital punishment's continued popularity in America, it is a useful case study in American bioethics as well.[2]

Physicians can play many roles in capital punishment, including preparing the prisoner for execution, supervising the execution, and pronouncing death, most of which are considered unethical.[3] A physician invented the guillotine, and physicians historically have regularly supervised executions, from the fictional naval surgeon who made sure the hanging of Melville's Billy Budd was "scientifically conducted"[4] to the physician who pinned a white circle over Gary Gilmore's heart as a target for the firing squad.[5] Another major role physicians can play is in determining which individuals should be excluded from the death penalty. One way is based on a medical determination of a person's ability to understand the death penalty and why it is being imposed.[6] In 2002 the U.S. Supreme Court expanded exclusionary criteria to include prohibiting execution of a person with a diagnosis of mental retardation.[7]

The physician's role in the death penalty is not only an issue of medical ethics but also inherently a political and legal issue, and in the American context it inevitably crosses over into both constitutional law and human rights principles. This is because by playing a role in an execution, the physician becomes an agent of the state and acts to further the state's death penalty policy. In terms of politics alone, the death penalty continues to have popular political support in the United States. National candidates have learned that the death penalty can become a symbol of a candidate's position on crime. Michael Dukakis, who opposed the death penalty, was brutalized as soft on crime in his presidential campaign. In the next presidential race, Bill Clinton took time off from his New Hampshire primary campaign to return to Arkansas to preside over the execution of Rickey Ray Rector. Rector was a violent criminal, and after murdering a police officer he shot himself in the head. He survived but was so severely brain damaged he was often described by journalists and others as mentally retarded.

Rector did not fit the medical definitions of mental retardation (because his condition did not manifest itself by age 18), but he was widely considered mentally retarded by the public. Nonetheless, the courts found him competent to stand trial and later competent to be executed, ruling that any clemency would have to come from Governor Clinton.[8] None was forthcoming, even though there is little doubt that Rector did not understand that he was going to be executed, as illustrated by the fact that just before his execution he saved the pecan pie from his last meal so he could eat it before he went to bed that night.[9] The public's sympathy was clearly with the families of Rector's victims rather than with Rector. After his execution the "soft on crime" label that had plagued Dukakis could not successfully be pinned on Clinton. As political consultant David Garth put it, Clinton "had someone put to death who had only part of a brain. You can't find them any tougher than that."[10]

Bill Clinton's decision to permit the execution of a severely brain-damaged prisoner was made more than a decade ago. Three years before that the U.S. Supreme Court had decided that it was not "cruel and unusual punishment" under the Eighth Amendment of the U.S. Constitution to execute a mentally retarded person. This was because mental retardation could be used as mitigating evidence in imposing a sentence, and there was "insufficient evidence" of a "national consensus against execution of the mentally retarded."[11] And in 1999, after the Texas Senate voted to bar the execution of the mentally retarded, then Governor George W. Bush voiced his opposition, saying, "That's up to juries to make those decisions . . . I like the law the way it is right now."[12]

In 2002, in *Atkins v. Virginia*, the U.S. Supreme Court reversed itself, ruling that the values of Americans had shifted in the past decade and that there now was a national consensus opposing execution of the mentally retarded. At issue in this case were questions central to universal human rights: moral progress and human dignity. Also implicated was the medical ethics issue of the role of medicine and physicians in the death penalty. The case involved Daryl Renard Atkins and the decision of the Commonwealth of Virginia to execute him.

The Crime

After a day spent drinking alcohol and smoking marijuana, William Jones and Daryl Renard Atkins abducted Eric Nesbitt outside a convenience store at midnight. They robbed him of the cash he was carrying and drove him in his pickup truck to an ATM, where they forced him to withdraw an additional $200. They then took him to a deserted area, where, ignoring his pleas, he was shot eight times (in the thorax, abdomen, arms, and legs) and killed. Each defendant testified that the other had fired the shots that killed Nesbitt, but the jury evidently believed it was Atkins who pulled the trigger. Jones was permitted to plead guilty to first-degree murder in exchange for his testimony against Atkins. The plea made Jones ineligible for the death sentence.

At the penalty phase of the trial, the defense relied solely on the testimony of Evan Nelson, a forensic psychologist who had evaluated Atkins before the trial and found him "mildly mentally retarded." His conclusion was based on interviews with Atkins and people who knew Atkins, a review of school and court records, and the measurement of his IQ as 59 on the Wechsler Adult Intelligence Scales Test. The jury sentenced Atkins to death, but the Virginia Supreme Court ordered a second sentencing hearing because the judge had used a misleading verdict form.

At the second hearing Nelson testified again. This time the state presented its own forensic psychologist, Stanton Samenow, who testified that Atkins was not mentally retarded but was of "average intelligence at least." The jury also heard testimony about the defendant's 16 earlier felony convictions for robbery, attempted robbery, abduction, use of a firearm, and maiming. Atkins was again sentenced to death, and the Virginia Supreme

Court affirmed the sentence.[13] Two judges dissented, noting that Samenow's opinion that Atkins possessed average intelligence was "incredulous as a matter of law" and concluding that "the imposition of the sentence of death upon a criminal defendant who has the mental age of a child between the ages of 9 and 12 is excessive." In their words, "It is indefensible to conclude that individuals who are mentally retarded are not to some degree less culpable for their criminal acts. By definition, such individuals have substantial limitations not shared by the general population. A moral and civilized society diminishes itself if its system of justice does not afford recognition and consideration of those limitations in a meaningful way."

The Punishment

The U.S. Supreme Court decided to hear the appeal not only "because of the gravity of the concerns expressed by the dissenters" but also "in light of the dramatic shift in the state legislative landscape that has occurred in the past 13 years." There was only one question before the Court: is the execution of a mentally retarded defendant cruel and unusual punishment prohibited by the Eighth Amendment of the U.S. Constitution? The Court had previously ruled that the Eighth Amendment, the text of which is "Excessive bail shall not be required, nor excessive fines imposed, nor cruel and unusual punishments inflicted," was based on the "precept of justice that punishment for crime should be graduated and proportioned to the offense."[14] Moreover, judgments about whether a punishment is excessive are to be made based not on the standards that prevailed when the Bill of Rights was adopted, but on those that currently prevail. As Chief Justice Earl Warren put it in a 1958 opinion: "The basic concept underlying the Eighth Amendment is nothing less than the dignity of man . . . The Amendment must draw its meaning from the evolving standards of decency that mark the progress of a maturing society."[15] A determination of existing standards is to be based on "objective factors to the maximum possible extent."

As noted, 13 years before *Atkins* the Court had concluded that executing a mentally retarded person did *not* violate the Eighth Amendment. The case involved the brain-damaged, mentally retarded Johnny Paul Penry, who was convicted of brutally raping, beating, and stabbing a woman to death using scissors. The Court found that only two states (Georgia and Maryland) had adopted laws banning the execution of a mentally retarded person. Even coupled with opinion polls showing large majorities of the public in Texas, Florida, and Georgia opposed executing the mentally retarded, and considering the 14 states that had no death penalty, this evidence was deemed "insufficient" to support the conclusion that there was "a national consensus" on the subject.[16]

But, as Justice John Paul Stevens, who wrote for the majority of the Court in the six-to-three *Atkins* opinion, noted, at least partially in response to the Court's *Penry* decision "state legislatures across the country began to address the issue." Since 1990 Kentucky, Tennessee, New Mexico, Arkansas (which passed its law in 1993, the year after Rector was executed), Colorado, Washington, Indiana, Kansas, New York, Nebraska, South Dakota, Arizona, Connecticut, Florida, Missouri, and North Carolina all have passed laws excluding persons with mental retardation from the death penalty. These 18 states do not represent a majority of the 38 death penalty states, but the Court decided "it is not so much the number of these States that is significant, but the consistency of the direction of change [especially] given the well-known fact that anticrime legislation is far more popular than legislation providing protection for persons guilty of violent crime."

The Court, noting further that no state had specifically authorized the execution of the mentally retarded, and that even in those states that still permitted it, only five people with IQs under 70 had actually been executed in the past 13 years, concluded: "The practice, therefore, has become truly unusual, and it is fair to say that a national consensus has developed against it." A footnote to this last sentence offers "additional evidence" that the states were reflecting "a much broader social and professional consensus," including: positions adopted by professional associations such as the American Psychological Association; Christian, Jewish, Muslim, and Buddhist traditions; the fact that the "world community" overwhelmingly disapproved of executing the mentally retarded; and state and national public opinion polls that demonstrated "a widespread consensus among Americans."[17]

Identifying the Mentally Retarded

Although it left the classification of individuals as mentally retarded to the individual states, the Court stressed the importance of applying the current clinical definition. In this regard it set forth both the definition of the American Association of Mental Retardation (AAMR) and that of the American Psychiatric Association (APA). The AAMR defines mental retardation as follows:

> Mental retardation refers to substantial limitations in present functioning. It is characterized by significantly subaverage intellectual functioning,

existing concurrently with related limitations in two or more of the following applicable adaptive skill areas: communication, self-care, home living, social skills, community use, self-direction, health and safety, functional academics, leisure, and work. Mental retardation manifests before age 18.

The APA's definition is substantially the same:

The essential feature of mental retardation is significantly subaverage general intellectual functioning (criterion A) that is accompanied by significant limitations in adaptive functioning in at least two of the following skill areas: communication, self-care, home living, social/ interpersonal skills, use of community resources, self-direction, functional academic skills, work, leisure, health, and safety (Criterion B). The onset must occur before age 18 years (Criterion C). . . . "Mild" mental retardation is typically used to describe people with an IQ level of 50–55 to approximately 70.

The Court concluded that although such "deficiencies do not warrant an exemption from criminal sanctions . . . they do diminish personal culpability." Specifically, the Court noted that the only two justifications for the death penalty, retribution and deterrence, could not be furthered by executing mentally retarded persons. In regard to retribution, the Court had earlier ruled that the death penalty must be reserved for exceptionally extreme acts. In this context the Court concluded, "If the culpability of the average murderer is insufficient to justify the most extreme sanction available to the State, the lesser culpability of the mentally retarded offender surely does not merit that form of retribution." As to deterrence, the Court found that the same mental deficiencies that make a person retarded make it "less likely that they can process the information of the possibility of execution as a penalty and, as a result, control their conduct based upon that information."

Dissenting opinions were written by Chief Justice William Rehnquist and Justice Antonin Scalia. The chief justice was particularly upset that the Court put any weight at all on "foreign laws, the views of professional and religious organizations, and opinion polls in reaching its conclusion," arguing that such sources, were irrelevant. Instead, the chief justice insisted that only two sources, "the work product of legislatures and sentencing jury determinations," are "objective indicia of contemporary values firmly supported by our precedents."

Justice Scalia opined, "Seldom has an opinion of this Court rested so obviously upon nothing but the personal views of its members." Scalia argued that there was no "national consensus" because only 18 of the 38 states that permitted capital punishment (or 47%) exempted the mentally retarded, and agreed with the Chief Justice that other sources of consensus were irrelevant. He concluded, moreover, that the definitions of mental retardation adopted by the AAMR and the APA would lead to "turning the process of capital trial into a game" because "the symptoms of this condition can readily be feigned," and "the capital defendant who feigns mental retardation risks nothing at all."

Moral Progress

Justice Scalia may be correct that the justices were voicing their personal opinions on the wrongness of executing a mentally retarded killer, but, as Justice Stevens noted, these are opinions shared by most of the world. We can also be skeptical of Kant's concept of moral progress. As philosopher Jonathan Glover has observed, "At the start of the twentieth century, reflective Europeans were able to believe in moral progress, and to see human viciousness and barbarism as in retreat. At the end of the century, [which has seen the results of technology in the service of the destructive side of human psychology] it is hard to be confident either about the moral law or about moral progress."[18] But moral progress has never been a steady march and human beings can become ashamed of their brutal behavior and take steps to try to prevent it. This is what the majority of the world's countries have done in abolishing the death penalty and what the U.S. Supreme Court has done in prohibiting the execution of mentally retarded killers. Shame is, after all, a major method of enforcing human rights norms around the world.[19]

Scalia is simply wrong, however, to try to read the "cruel and unusual" injunction in the Eighth Amendment as the citizens of the United States would have read it in 1791, when it was written. I also think the majority of the Court is correct to look beyond the shores of the United States to what is going on in the rest of the world. We are all members of the same species, we all have human dignity, and we all share the same planet and future. We do not steadily progress to be better people, but we should not aspire to limit the boundaries of our national morality to those of an age in which none of us live and in which almost none of our globalizing, and potentially brutalizing, technology existed.

The Court's opinion immediately evoked contrasting responses concerning its impact on the broader question of the death penalty itself. One view is that it can be seen as part of an inexorable, if slow, moral progress march toward abolition of the death penalty.[20] In this view, the United States has become, as the Court noted, increasingly out of step with the democracies of the world. In a post 9/11 world, we not only line up with countries in the "axis of evil" in maintaining our death penalty, we also make it less likely that any European country will extradite suspected terrorists to the United States because of the possibility that they will face the death penalty.

The contrasting view holds that the public's support for the death penalty only erodes when it is applied in ways that seem unjust and unfair, such as against the mentally retarded or those whose lawyers literally fell asleep during their trials. To the extent that these cases are moved outside the realm of the death penalty, those that remain may seem fair and just, making the death penalty itself more likely rather than less likely to survive.[21]

In the two years since *Atkins* only a handful of prisoners have left death row as a result of a finding of mental retardation, although the issue has been more often addressed prior to trial.[22] Because the Court did not tell states how to determine the question of mental retardation, each state has had to adopt its own procedures. Some have opted to let the judge decide; some, including Virginia, will use a jury to make the determination; and others have not yet decided how to proceed. The Court has also accepted a case on executing 16- and 17-year-old offenders, and it seems likely that the Court will find this practice unconstitutional as well, on the same basis on which *Atkins* was decided. International law, including the Convention on the Rights of the Child, supports such a conclusion.

The Role of Physicians

In May 2002 the American Medical Association "strongly reaffirmed" its opposition to physician participation in execution, as outlined in its often updated ethical statement on capital punishment. It is likely that as a result of the *Atkins* opinion more convicted killers will want to be labeled mentally retarded and more physicians and psychologists will be asked to become involved in mental retardation evaluations. Using one's medical skills as an agent of the state to help make a mentally ill prisoner "fit" for execution is, of course, a perversion of medicine—in the same category as monitoring the health of a person who is being tortured.[23] But applying medical criteria to possibly exclude someone from the death penalty on the basis of mental retardation need not be classified as unethical medical work that puts the physician in the service of the state's death machinery. Because the medical criteria used to diagnose mental retardation are so vague, however, it may be difficult for physicians to act in any but a political manner in this context, at least in borderline cases. Terms such as "substantial limitations" and "significantly subaverage," for example, are inherently subjective. I.Q. tests are notoriously misleading, and there is no blood test or other objective clinical test to determine mental retardation.[24] On the other hand, Scalia's fears about gamesmanship are overblown because mental retardation is a lifelong developmental disability and an "individual cannot fake school records or other indicators of historically significant subaverage performance" before age 18.[25] Nonetheless, physicians could understandably decline to participate in mental retardation evaluations, even before trial, arguing that their participation in any phase of a proceeding that could end in the death penalty lends legitimacy to capital punishment and thus makes medicine complicit in executions.

At this juncture in the death penalty debate, medical ethics and physicians are now front and center. This is because the primary factor that is saving the death penalty itself from being declared cruel and unusual punishment is execution by lethal injection. This method of killing medicalizes capital punishment and makes it seem much more benign and certainly less violent than hanging, electrocution, gassing, or the firing squad.

As the Court made clear in finding the execution of the mentally retarded unconstitutional, the continued ability of the justices to support the constitutionality of the death penalty rests on its approval by public opinion. Public opinion is likely to be influenced by the opinion of physicians and medical organizations. The states that continue to use the death penalty have appropriated medical techniques and knowledge to make it appear humane. As Scott Turow has observed, the execution chamber in Illinois "remains a solemn spot, with the sterile feel of an operating theatre in a hospital. The execution gurney, where the lethal injection is administered, is covered by a crisp sheet and might even be mistaken for an examining table."[26] My colleagues Joan LeGraw and Michael Grodin seem correct to conclude that because of the centrality of lethal injection to executions, the medical profession now bears a "collective responsibility" for the continuation of capital punishment, and physicians should therefore do what they can to eliminate lethal injection as a method of execution, whether or not they personally support capital punishment.[27] In capital punishment in the United States, medical ethics has become an integral component of human rights and constitutional law.

II

. . . .

BIOETHICS AND HEALTH LAW

7

. . . .

Conjoined Twins

Many, if not most, bioethical dilemmas wind up in America's courtrooms. Ardent disputes arise at the beginning and end of life, and these have been most emblematic in the cases of abortion and physician-assisted suicide. American courts have been much more successful in resolving continuing bioethical conflicts in the latter than in the former. Nonetheless, that both made their way to the U.S. Supreme Court surprised almost no one. And although America is unique in its persistent appeal to judges to resolve bioethical issues, it is not alone in looking to judges for help in their resolution. In this sense, international bioethics is mimicking American bioethics by crossing over into the territory of health law. This chapter introduces judicial decision making in the most extreme context: the separation of conjoined twins in cases in which surgery will either kill one of the twins or could kill both. The issue of separating conjoined twins forces us to confront the limits of law at the limits of life.

Conjoined twin surgery almost always involves infants, but in the summer of 2003 the world watched first in fascination and then in sorrow as surgeons in Singapore attempted the world's first separation of adult twins joined at the head. Ladan and Laleh Bijani, from Iran, were 29 years old at the time, and neither survived the two-day surgery to separate them.[1] All conjoined twin separations raise two central issues: can separation be successful for at least one twin (and, of course, what does "successful" mean?), and, if so, can informed consent be obtained?

In young children, like the case of Jodie and Mary Attard, which will be discussed in detail later, the issue of consent revolves primarily around the question of whether the parents are the proper people to grant or with-hold it. In the case of the adult Bijanis, only they had the legal and moral authority to consent. An ethics committee was set up to review their deci-sion and seems to have concluded that the twins were determined to undergo the procedure. There are some critical questions—and all the facts of what actually happened in this case have not yet been made public. Most central is the question of whether both twins had to agree, or whether either one of them could have demanded to be separated from the other. All press reports indicated that both Bijanis wanted the surgery, but it is unclear whether any attempt was made to interview them separately (the Farrelly brothers' movie, *Stuck on You*, suggests how this could be done). It seems reasonable to assume that they both did want the surgery. Nonethe-less, informed consent would have required that the twins appreciate the extremely high risk of death and serious brain injury. Press reports indi-cated that the twins were told that the risk of death to each of them was 50 percent and that they accepted this risk.

The central ethical question was whether a surgical separation that involved such a high mortality risk was medically acceptable, given that the procedure was not medically necessary for the health or life of either twin but was done primarily to improve their quality of life by permitting each twin to live independently. This is an extremely difficult ethical ques-tion, although bioethicists who have commented on it have almost uniformly said simply that if the physicians believed it was medically reasonable, then whether to proceed should have been left up to the twins. The working assumption seems to be that living as a conjoined twin is so obviously oppressive to each twin that a desire to be separated makes perfect sense. The physicians, nonetheless, have mostly said that they proceeded because the twins insisted. Even if the state of being a conjoined twin is pathologi-cal, because the surgery is extreme and dangerous it should only be at-tempted with the informed and persistent consent of both twins.

This logic is circular and simply begs the question of whether a sepa-ration is medically reasonable. This turns on the probability of success and what is meant by success. It seems reasonable to assume that in the view of the twins, success would have been the ability to live independently with

full brain function. If there really was a 50 percent chance of such an outcome, then the twins should have been able to authorize their surgeons to
proceed. But what if the real odds were only 10 percent or 1 percent? What
is the statistical cutoff at which point the operation becomes more like
physician-assisted suicide than surgery? And given the fact that such an
operation had never even been attempted, is any statistical estimate of
success misleading?

During the operation itself the surgeons believed that it would make
sense to pause and perform the separation in phases because of the difficulty detaching the bone and controlling the circulation. Nonetheless, the
surgeons acceded to the wishes of the relatives to continue the procedure
no matter what the risk of massive bleeding. As Ben Carson, a neurosur-
geon from Johns Hopkins who was on the surgical team, put it, "At that
point I felt like a person heading into a dark jungle to hunt a hungry tiger
with no gun." That is not a good way for a surgeon to feel and is reminis-
cent of a statement by the surgeon who performed the world's first human
heart transplant, Christiaan Barnard. When asked if he thought his patient
was brave, he said no. In his words, "For a dying man it is not a difficult
decision. . . . If a lion chases you to the bank of a river filled with croco-
diles, you will leap into the water convinced you have a chance to swim to
the other side. But you would never accept such odds if there were no
lion." Both surgeons, it would seem, decided that a central issue was how
they felt about proceeding, not how the patients might feel. This may be
unfair to Carson, who has since been appointed to the President's Council
on Bioethics. About two months after the operation, he explained the initial decision to do the operation:

> They were going to eventually get [the operation] done. That became
> very clear to me. Now I must say, you know, going into it, I felt like
> many other people, being stuck together, it's not that bad . . . you
> can get by. Come on, get over it. But after I met them I understood
> . . . they were extremely vivacious, very intelligent, but quite de-
> pressed. And it became clear as I talked to them the reason for the
> depression. They had very, very different aspirations in terms of
> where their lives would go, and yet they couldn't get there because
> they were stuck together, because every decision was a committee
> decision, even going to the bathroom . . . they said to me they
> couldn't stand it and that they'd rather die than to spend another
> day attached. I felt a little better about my decision to participate
> but still recognizing that it was going to be an extraordinarily diffi-
> cult and challenging situation.[2]

A coroner later returned a verdict of medical misadventure, which cleared the physicians of any criminal wrongdoing, and found that the twins gave their informed consent to the surgery. At the coroner's inquest, Carson testified candidly that if he had known at the time what he knew now, he would have paused the operation when severe bleeding began, even though the pause itself carried grave risks.[3] Much more commonly in cases involving conjoined twins, legal questions are raised and dealt with before the surgery.

Conjoined twins are oddities and have long been the subject of scientific exhibits, medical study, and human curiosity. They are unusual, even bizarre, and usually are very young. The Lakeberg twins, for example, were born about a decade ago in Illinois. The hospital in which they were born determined that there was no chance for either to survive and that the best thing to do was let them both die. Children's Hospital of Philadelphia saw it differently and offered to try to separate them. So the parents took the children to Philadelphia. One died during surgery, which they had more or less known would happen, and the other died a year later. The procedure cost about $2 million.[4] The decision to proceed was made by the parents, and it is elementary U.S. law that parents make the difficult treatment decisions for their children.[5]

Ten years earlier, at that same hospital in Philadelphia, there was a similar case. Dr. C. Everett Koop, the former U.S. Surgeon General, was the surgeon and was afraid he might be sued for killing one of the children during a separation operation.[6] He asked the local district attorney what to do. The parents of the conjoined twins, who shared a heart, were Jewish, so they talked to their rabbi. The nurses were Catholic, so they talked to their priest. The priest said one could fit separation of conjoined twins into the principle of double effect (in a sense, what the U.S. Supreme Court said when it determined it was lawful to prescribe enough drugs to keep a patient out of pain, even if the drugs hastened the patient's death). To oversimplify, the double effect is that if an act has both a good and an evil effect, as long as one does not intend the evil effect, but only the good effect, and the good effect does not come directly from the evil effect, and there is proportionality between the good effect and the evil effect, the act is licit. The priest argued that although separating the twins would kill one twin, she would not be killed intentionally or directly, but rather she would die indirectly from the legitimate treatment of the other twin. I do not find that terribly persuasive, but the double effect worked for them.

The rabbi, I think, was more helpful, and as will be discussed, the two examples that rabbinical scholars found useful were used by all three judges in the Attard case. The first involves a caravan in the middle of the desert that is attacked by bandits. The bandits demand a particular person, or they will destroy the entire caravan. The caravan can send out the person demanded, even though they know the bandits are going to kill him, because the person has been "designated for death." In the other example, two people parachute from a plane, and only one of their parachutes opens. The unfortunate parachuter grabs the leg of the person whose parachute opened to try to save himself. It would be moral for the man with the open parachute to kick the other man off if the parachute was not strong enough for both to survive, because the person whose parachute did not open was "designated for death." And so in the Philadelphia case the argument followed that the weaker of the two conjoined twins, the twin who was less likely to survive, was designated for death, and therefore it was morally acceptable (although not required) to do the separation operation.

The Conjoined Twins from Gozo

The conjoined twins who were the subject of two British court decisions were Jodie and Mary (not their real names), the children of Michaelangelo and Rina Attard of the Maltese island of Gozo.[7] The couple, who were Roman Catholic, came to England for medical care at about five months gestation, and the conjoined twins were born on August 8, 2000. The children were joined at the pelvis, their spinal columns on the same axis, with each having two arms and two legs. The physicians saw no hope of the twins surviving for more than a year if they remained joined but believed that if Mary (the weaker of the two, whose continued survival depended on sharing Jodie's circulatory system) was separated from Jodie, Mary would die, but Jodie would survive and do well. The parents refused to consider authorizing the separation on the basis that it was wrong to choose between the lives of their two innocent children and also contrary to their religious beliefs. Physicians have historically honored the wishes of parents in cases like this.[8] In this case, however, the physicians abandoned this medical ethics stance and decided to go to court to obtain authority to proceed with the separation over the objections of the parents.

In the United States the decision of the parents would be final unless the physicians or the state could persuade a judge that this was a case of child neglect.[9] In England the law is different: once a case is placed before a judge, the judge must decide what the "welfare" or "best interests" of the child requires by exercising "an independent and objective judgment." The parents' wishes are just one piece of evidence to be considered in making this determination. The trial court judge concluded that separation was in the best interests of both children and that separation was not a case of killing Mary, but one of passive euthanasia, in which her food and hydration would be withdrawn (by clamping off her blood supply from Jodie). The parents and the official solicitor appointed to represent Mary appealed.

Each of the three judges on the appeals panel issued a separate opinion, as is customary in English courts. Although all the judges agreed with the trial court judge that the separation should be done, none agreed with the legal reasoning of the trial court, and none of the judges fully agreed with the others' legal reasoning.[10] There were many reasons for this, including the unprecedented nature of the dispute itself, reliance on analogies that did not quite fit, and a strong desire to authorize physicians to do what they thought best for their newborn patients.

Justice Alan Ward

Lord Justice Alan Ward begins his analysis by noting that this "truly is a unique case" that "in a nutshell" involves killing the weaker twin, Mary (who would not have been viable had she been a singleton) to "give Jodie a life which will be worthwhile." Ward describes the physical condition of the twins in detail, quoting from physician reports that document, among other things, that Jodie has "an anatomically normal brain, heart, lungs and liver," that she is expected to be of "normal intelligence," and that she "appears to be a bright little girl." Mary, on the other hand, is described by physicians as "severely abnormal," having a "primitive" brain, a very poorly functioning heart, and an absence of lung tissue. Ward concludes that Mary is incapable of surviving separately: "She lives on borrowed time, all of which is borrowed from Jodie. It is a debt she can never repay." He notes that separation will cause Mary's death (which the physicians believe will be quick and painless) and that a heart–lung transplant for Mary (again, according to the physicians) is not an option.

Justice Ward then turns to the question of why the court is involved at all, noting that although "every instinct of the medical team has been to save life where it can be saved," it would have been "perfectly acceptable" for the medical team and hospital to have respected the parental refusal even though this would have resulted in the death of both twins. But seeking court authorization for surgery is also acceptable in Ward's view because "here sincere professionals could not allay a collective medical conscience and see children in their care die when they know one was capable of being saved. They could not proceed in the absence of parental consent. The only arbiter of that sincerely held difference of opinion is the court. Deciding disputed matters of life and death is surely and pre-eminently a matter for a court of law to judge."

In analyzing existing law, Ward strongly disagrees with the trial court, saying that it is "utterly fanciful" to classify the operation as "an omission," and that there is no way that killing Mary can be "in Mary's best interests." Instead, he concludes that the only proper legal path when there is a conflict of interest between conjoined twins is "to choose the lesser of two evils." Ward condemns the parents' refusal to choose life for Jodie in dramatic terms: "In my judgment, parents who are placed on the horns of such a terrible dilemma simply have to choose the lesser of their inevitable loss. If a family at the gates of a concentration camp were told they might free one of their children but if no choice were made both would die, compassionate parents with equal love for their twins would elect to save the stronger and see the weak one destined for death pass through the gates." He goes on to say, "my heart bleeds for them. But . . . it is I who must now make the decision."

The decision, of course, seems to have been dictated by the description of the condition of the two twins, but it still must be legally justified. Ward does this by accusing Mary of killing Jodie, thus making a decision to kill Mary justifiable homicide, a case of "quasi self-defense": "Mary may have a right to life, but she has little right to be alive. She is alive because . . . she [parasitically] sucks the lifeblood out of Jodie. If Jodie could speak, she would surely protest, 'Stop it, Mary, you're killing me.'" Ward concludes that the physicians have a legal duty to Jodie that gives them an obligation to act, and that "doctors cannot be denied a right of choice if they are under a duty to choose."

Justice Robert Brooke

Lord Justice Robert Brooke horrified the parents when, in open court, he looked at pictures of the twins and asked "What is this creature in the eyes of the law?"[11] His opinion, however, is more analytical. He agrees with Ward's family law analysis but believes more is required to persuasively conclude that the operation that would kill Mary is lawful. The official solicitor, who opposed the separation, suggested nonetheless that the court might wish to develop new law that permitted such an operation if it was "proportionate and necessary" and "approved in advance by the court." Brooke essentially adopts this as a reasonable approach, and much of his opinion explores the legal doctrine of necessity.

The major case he examines is *Regina v. Dudley and Stephens*, a memorable 1884 case that involved shipwreck and survival on the high seas by means of murder and cannibalism.[12] A crew of four was sailing the yacht *Mignonette* from England to Australia when their ship came apart in a storm in the South Atlantic 2000 miles from land. The crew escaped in a lifeboat with only two cans of turnips. After 19 days the three senior members of the crew killed 17-year-old Richard Parker, the youngest and weakest member of the crew, and ate him in order to survive. They later explained that the point of killing him before he died naturally was to be able to drink his blood.[13] After being rescued and returned to England, they were arrested and tried for murder, a charge they did not deny. Their defense was "necessity." The British courts rejected this defense, noting among other things that the boy did not threaten the rest of the crew and that the law could not justify choosing the "unoffending and unresisting boy" to die, "the weakest, the youngest, the most unresisting. . . . Was it more necessary to kill him than one of the grown men? The answer must be 'No.'"

Although so far rejected by British law, Brooke suggests there may be circumstances in which the necessity defense should be allowed. He gives several examples. The first is the case of a mountain climber who must cut the rope holding another climber who has fallen, otherwise both will perish. The next is the sinking of the passenger ferry *Herald of Free Enterprises* near Zeebrugge, Belgium, in which almost 200 passengers drowned. An army corporal said that he and dozens of other people were in the water near the foot of a rope ladder and all in danger of drowning. Their route to safety was blocked by a young man on the ladder who was paralyzed with fear and unable to move. Eventually the corporal ordered that the man be pushed off the ladder so that the others could climb to safety. As mentioned earlier, two other examples had been suggested by a rabbi who counseled a Jewish couple considering a similar operation on their conjoined twins (who shared a single heart) in Philadelphia in 1977, and Brooke describes these as well.

Many more legal authorities are quoted at length, but ultimately Justice Brooke concludes that the *Dudley* cannibalism case is distinguishable because neither of the objections to the necessity defense presented in *Dudley* are applicable to the twins case (who can judge this sort of necessity, and how can the comparative value of lives be measured?) because "Mary is, sadly, self-designated for a very early death." He also thinks there is no danger of the necessity defense being misused by physicians in other conjoined twins cases because "there will be in practically every case the opportunity for the doctors to place the relevant facts before a court for approval (or otherwise) before the operation is attempted."

Justice Robert Walker

Lord Justice Robert Walker opens his opinion by describing this case as "tragic" and "unprecedented anywhere in the world." Although conjoined twins are unique, Walker insists that "there is no longer any place in the legal textbooks, any more than there is in the medical textbooks, for expressions (such as 'monster') which are redolent of superstitious horror. Such disparagingly emotive language should never be used to describe a human being, however disabled or dysmorphic." He nonetheless concludes that continued life joined to Jodie would "confer no benefit [on Mary] but would be to her disadvantage." Walker agrees with Brooke that the question of whether Mary can be lawfully killed for Jodie's sake rests on the issues of intention and necessity. Like Brooke, he reviews a series of analogies, but unlike him, Walker concludes that "there is no helpful analogy or parallel to . . . this case."

Ultimately, Walker determines that the physicians owe conflicting duties to the twins. Nonetheless, he believes the dilemma does not involve choosing "the relative worth of two human beings," but rather "undertaking surgery without which neither life will have the bodily integrity (or wholeness) which is its due." He believes having her "bodily integrity," if only for a few seconds, is a benefit to Mary. He concludes that physicians would separate the twins not with the intent of killing Mary, but with the intent of making each twin whole and acting in the best interests of both. What seems to persuade Walker the most, however, is the testimony of the physicians: "Highly skilled and conscientious doctors believe that the best course, in the interests of both twins, is to undertake elective surgery in order to separate them and save Jodie."

The Surgery

Controversy continued after the opinion was delivered over which of two surgical teams, the one with more experience or the one that brought the case to court, should perform the surgery.[14] It was finally performed by the less experienced team after the opinion was issued.[15] The surgeons involved later told the press that they, like Koop in Philadelphia, were worried about being prosecuted for murder for killing Mary, and that is why they sought court approval.[16] The surgeons continued to believe that separation was in the best interests of both twins (although it caused Mary's death). When the final blood vessels that connected the twins were cut in the separation operation, an act that would result in the death of Mary, the two lead surgeons said they cut the blood vessels together, in silence, and with "great respect." The coroner recorded a narrative verdict, stating simply that Mary died "following surgery separating her from her conjoined twin, which surgery was permitted by an order of the High Court, confirmed by the Court of Appeal."[17] Jodie (whose real name is Gracie) returned home to Gozo to live with her parents, although she will require extensive surgery over the next five years or more. Mary (whose real name was Rosie) was buried on Gozo.[18] The parents had another girl, whom they named Rosie in memory of Gracie's sister.[19]

Problems with the Legal Analysis

It is easy to see why all the judges involved characterized this case as "unique" and hoped that it would not set a precedent. This is because the case seems not to have been decided on the law (which most of the judges found of little help), but on an intuitive judgment that the state of being a conjoined twin is a disease and that separation is the indicated treatment for it, at least if it affords one of the twins a chance to live. The judges identified strongly with the physicians and had little empathy with the parents or their religious beliefs. I think these factors led each judge to make problematic legal statements.

Justice Ward is the hardest on the parents, using the *Sophie's Choice* analogy of a parent at the gates of a concentration camp. The Nazi physician in charge of selecting who is to go to the gas chambers immediately and who can do labor or be used in medical experiments tells Sophie that both her children will be killed if she does not choose one to save.[20] Justice Ward insists that a parent in this situation "must" choose. Sophie, of course, did choose, although she ultimately lost both children to the Nazis and killed herself because she was unable to live with her coerced decision.

Ward's *Sophie's Choice* analogy, at the heart of his analysis, is troubling in at least two respects. The first is his conclusion that parents must choose which child to die when only one can be saved. We would not condemn a parent for making this terrible choice, but neither should we condemn a parent for refusing to make it. For example, if a father jumps from a burning plane holding two children, one in each arm, and on the way down he begins to lose his grip on both and knows that he will drop them both if he does not drop one to save the other, we would not fault him for dropping one. Neither, I believe, should we fault a parent for refusing to choose and instead trying to hang on to both children for as long as possible. Second, and more disturbing with respect to the concentration camp example, is the question of who the judge thinks plays the role of the

Nazi physician. Ward concludes that it is the British physicians who "should be given the right of choice," but he also seems to place himself in that role, saying, "it is I who must now make the decision." Of course, Ward is not choosing to kill both twins, and perhaps he sees nature as the Nazis, and himself as Sophie. Nonetheless, it is unsettling to see a British judge rely on what might be termed "concentration camp ethics" to reach his decision.

Justice Ward is not much stronger on the law. He insists, for example, that the law requires him to do what is in the best interests of the children, and that British law prohibits the use of the doctrine of substituted judgment (determining what an incompetent person would decide if capable of making a decision). Nonetheless, his primary argument turns out to be basically a substituted judgment one: in colorful language he likens Mary to a parasite who is "poisoning" Jodie and sucking out her "lifeblood." He knows what Jodie would decide if she could decide: "If Jodie could speak, she would surely protest, 'Stop it, Mary, you're killing me.'" But the problem with using substituted judgment for very young children is that we have no way to know what they would say and tend to speculate on the basis of our own adult values. For example, Jodie could equally well say to her identical and attached twin that "I love you as myself and will do everything, including sacrificing my life, to keep you alive as long as possible." Likewise, Mary might reasonably say to Jodie, "You are my identical twin, and I love you, so I'm willing to die so you can live since this is the only chance there is for my genes to be transmitted to the next generation." Each twin might also, of course, consider the other twin a part of "me" that should not be amputated. Any of these hypotheses is plausible, but made up dramatic monologues cannot substitute for legal analysis. With adult conjoined twins, like the Bijanis, we can, of course, talk to them directly, and they can make decisions like these themselves.

Justice Brooke's opinion is also problematic because he does not properly interpret the analogies he uses. His reliance on the necessity defense, for example, is based almost exclusively on the two analogies he describes that were reportedly used by the rabbi who counseled a Jewish couple similarly situated in Philadelphia in 1977: the men jumping from the burning plane, and the caravan surrounded by bandits. In each, the necessity defense is said to be appropriate because the person killed was "designated for death," a phrase Brooke adopts as his primary justification for killing Mary to save Jodie. In fact, he goes further, concluding "Mary is, sadly, self-designated for a very early death." There are two problems with this conclusion. First, Mary was not designated for anything, she was simply born and survived. But even the simple "designated for death" label may not be a proper reading of the two analogies.

The description of the two analogies was taken by the justices from an article I wrote in 1987, and I used a 1977 newspaper report as my own source.[21] More important than what might have been lost in the retelling, however, is that expert commentary on these examples has since been published, and the justices seemed unaware of it.

A leading U.S. rabbinical authority, Rabbi J. David Bleich, has written that these two analogies are not properly characterized as "designated for death" cases.[22] Instead, the parachutist example is better thought of as a "pursuer" case, in which the parachutist is justified in kicking off the man clinging to his leg because his intentional actions will otherwise kill the parachutist. In the second example, Rabbi Bleich argues the caravan is justified in turning over the named person only if that person is guilty of having committed some crime; if the person is innocent, he may not be turned over to a certain death. It has been suggested elsewhere that a group similarly situated could lawfully agree to use a random device, like drawing straws, to pick a person to be sacrificed for the good of the group.[23] Rabbi Bleich does nonetheless offer Justice Brooke another possible justification for his conclusion. Bleich believes that there may be exceptional circumstances in which one conjoined twin can be ethically judged a pursuer of the other: "If the heart can be shown to belong to one twin exclusively, the second is, in effect, a parasite . . . [and having] no claim to the heart, is then quite literally a pursuer." Pursuers must be stopped before they kill, and self-defense would have provided Brooke with a much sounder rationale for his conclusion than did the "designated for death" approach.

Finally, Justice Walker's opinion is, I think, most notable in trying (but failing) to consider the conjoined twins as simultaneously a single entity and two persons. Walker wants to discourage the use of terms like "monster" and "creature" to describe conjoined twins. Nonetheless, he speaks of them not as one entity, but as two separate "innocent children" and believes the "court must consider the welfare of each." The problem is that once the twins are separated verbally, it is only a matter of time before they will be separated surgically. Walker sees these conjoined twins as a serious, lethal anomaly that must be medically corrected so that at least one of the twins can appear normal. In this regard Walker seems correct in concluding, "in truth there is no helpful analogy or parallel to the current situation." He thus seems to find the condition of being a conjoined twin itself adequate justification for separation, at least when one could live if the other were killed. That is why he can conclude, with the physicians, the trial court judge, and Justice Brooke, that separation would be in the best interests of both children. Stated another way, three of the four judges who heard this case believed Mary would be better off dead than continuing to live for a few months as a conjoined twin.

Lessons

Perhaps the most important lesson of the case of Jodie and Mary is that there are severe limits to judicial decision making in complex life and death cases. The most important shortcoming of these judicial decisions is that they do not rest on any legal principle. That is why if an identical case were to be presented today to the Great Ormond Street Hospital for Children, the physicians could, under the rationale of this case (and contrary to its conclusion), decide to follow the wishes of the parents and let both twins die. The conclusion of Justice Ward that it would have been "perfectly acceptable" for the physicians to decide either way must be wrong: if Mary is a pursuer who is killing Jodie, saving Jodie's life (and others in her situation) by killing Mary must be mandatory for the physicians. The court's ruling that physicians can do whatever they think is best (with the court's prior approval) is no legal rule at all. It is also untrue that there will almost always be ample time to seek court review in cases like this.[24]

Closely related is the question of the court's role in similar cases: is it to determine whether a particular course of action, chosen by both parents and physicians, is legally permissible, or is it to determine if a particular medical intervention is required by law? The first role seems reasonable, but the second seems justified only in cases in which failure to act (on the part of either parents or physicians) is child neglect. In this regard, had Jodie been a singleton, the parents might well have been justified in refusing to consent to three or more years of heroic surgical procedures with an uncertain outcome on the basis that they did not believe the burdens of these interventions could be justified by the expected outcome even if the physician believed the operations were in her best interests.[25]

My own view is that in this case it would have been better for the physicians not to have sought court intervention, and if they did, for the trial court to have refused to hear this case and to have instructed the physicians that they must obtain the consent of the parents before separating the twins. I would have liked to see the parents agree to the separation (because giving Jodie a chance to live at the cost of cutting Mary's life short does seem the lesser of two evils), but I don't believe the case for separation was so strong that it demanded that the moral authority to make the decision about the medical treatment of their children should have been taken away from the parents.

Conjoined twin separations that necessitate killing one twin to save the other really do push us to the limits of the law. And at that limit, judges tend to reach technologically constructed decisions mediated by experts—in this case physicians, and in the Bijani case new image-guided surgery technology.

We seem to literally believe that physicians should be able to make life and death decisions for us, and if they want to go to court, that is fine, because courts almost uniformly bless whatever physicians want to do.[26] How has medicine gotten such a hold on the judiciary that judges authorize and promote almost anything physicians want done, even if the judges must use analogies to the Nazis, people jumping out of airplanes, and monsters to authorize physicians to do what they want to do? I think it is because of the power that physicians have over our lives, the power science and medical technology have over our lives, and our hope that medicine and science will become even more powerful and help us achieve virtual immortality. And if virtual immortality on earth is our goal, medicine quite naturally replaces religion in our lives.

It also seems to follow that if physicians hold the key to immortality, then physicians (not judges) should determine what is criminal and what is not in the medical realm: medicine, surgery, research, and whatever else might keep us alive longer. Almost every court, whether considering abortion, separating conjoined twins, or terminal sedation, has adopted the view that it is at least a rebuttable presumption that physicians' practices should be honored. The bottom line is that what physicians think is the right thing to do has consistently been legally protected by judges. In this sense, health law has incorporated the pragmatic medical ethics of physicians, especially surgeons, and made it de facto a part of health law itself. It is thus not an overstatement to conclude that good medical ethics is good law, as we have previously seen in documents as diverse as the Nuremberg Code, the protocols to the Geneva Conventions, and Comment 14 on the international right to health. The next chapter deals with more routine matters of medical practice and medical ethics from the legal perspective as mediated by health care institutions and organizations, patient rights.

8

. . . .

Patient Rights

The physician–philosopher head of President George W. Bush's Bioethics Council, Leon Kass, wrote in 1991, and repeated in 2002, that although "bioethics is where the action is," the action itself is "mostly talk" and abstract theory, with little impact on actual physician practice: "Though originally intended to improve our deeds, the reigning practice of ethics, if truth be told, has, at best, improved our speech."[1] There is, of course, some truth to this overgeneralization, and it helps explain why patients and their advocates turn to law rather than bioethics to improve health care and patient safety. Both modern bioethics and the modern patient rights movement can be seen as reactions to medical paternalism— but, in America at least, the patient rights movement has been considerably more powerful. Rights talk has even been seen as a substitute for a national health program, perhaps under the theory that rights in health care are much less expensive than are rights to health care.[2] American law on patient rights is almost exclusively state law, and federal regulations, like the HIPAA medical record privacy regulations, are aberrations to this rule.[3] Nonetheless, it is well worth considering whether a national patient bill of rights might help us move more decisively from bioethics talk to action in health care.

President Bill Clinton first proposed a national patient bill of rights in his 1998 State of the Union address. The president said, "You have the right to know all your medical options, not just the cheapest. You have the right to choose the doctor you want for the care you need. You have the right to emergency room care, wherever and whenever you need it. You have the right to keep your medical records confidential." The president's proposal was a follow-up to his announcement that he would codify the recommendations of his Commission on Consumer Protection and Quality in the Health Care Industry into a federal law. This idea followed proposals from almost every state legislature, the American Association of Health Plans, and an ad hoc group of nonprofit HMOs to provide Americans enrolled in health plans with new protections. The last time patient rights had been prominent was during the early 1970s.

Patient Rights in the 1970s

As Paul Starr has chronicled, in the early 1970s the movement to establish a right to health care was joined (some would say eclipsed) by a movement to establish rights in health care.[4] The right to health care demands federal legislation and financing, but rights in health care are almost always made obligatory by the courts.

The most important of all patient rights, the right to informed consent (better termed "informed choice"), was established in a series of court opinions in 1972, and soon thereafter became a principle of American bioethics as well. In these opinions the courts for the first time made it clear that the law would treat the doctor–patient relationship as a fiduciary, or trust, relationship, not an arms-length business relationship. The nature of this relationship is that a sick person (a patient) seeks the help of a specially educated and experienced professional, who is licensed by the state to practice medicine and whose unequal status vis-à-vis the patient requires the physician to assume certain legal obligations to the patient. These obligations are inherent in the doctor–patient relationship and require that before the physician elicits the patient's consent to treatment, the physician must provide the patient with some basic information so that the patient (not the physician) can make the final decision about whether to proceed. This information includes a description of the proposed treatment, anticipated risks and benefits, alternatives (including no treatment) and their risks and benefits, the probability of success, and the major anticipated problems of recuperation.[5]

All this seems pretty commonsensical more than 30 years later, but it was revolutionary at the time (informed consent had been legally required only for experimentation prior to these opinions). Perhaps the most important thing about the development of informed consent in the therapeutic setting, however, is that it was not a concept that had been promoted or embraced by medicine or medical ethics: it had to be imposed on medicine by law. American bioethics is often more pragmatic than principled—and to the extent it has principles, these principles are mostly drawn from American law. The primary example is autonomy.

Informed consent was followed by other developments designed to enhance the autonomy of patients. Autonomy, or liberty (sometimes reduced simply to choice), is, of course, the fundamental American value, and it is somewhat remarkable that medicine had been insulated from it until the 1970s. It is not surprising, then, that patient rights based on autonomy quickly became the norm. In early 1973, for example, the U.S. Supreme Court issued what is still its most important bioethics-related decision, *Roe v. Wade*,[6] discussed in some detail in Chapter 10. In this case the Court determined that pregnant women have a constitutional right of privacy that includes their right to continue or terminate a pregnancy in the absence of the state's ability to demonstrate a compelling interest in protecting fetal life. The case also stands for the proposition that the constitution limits state interference in the doctor–patient relationship.[7]

Also in early 1973, the American Hospital Association issued its own version of a patient bill of rights. Although the 12-point bill was vague and general, it was also historic and included many basic concepts of patient rights, such as the right to respectful care, the right to complete diagnosis and prognosis information, the right to informed consent, the right to refuse treatment, the right to refuse to participate in experiments, the right to privacy and confidentiality, and the right to a reasonable response to a request for services.

In an era when the routine use of medical technology came to be more important than its effectiveness in meeting patient needs, courts were called upon to enhance the power of patients. For example, in a series of cases, beginning in 1976 with the case of Karen Ann Quinlan and culminating in 1997 with the physician-assisted suicide cases, the courts affirmed the competent patient's right to refuse any medical treatment, including life-sustaining treatment. Moreover, patients, while competent, were authorized by statute to designate another person (a health care agent or proxy) to make treatment decisions for them if they became incompetent, and could make their wishes known in advance through a living will.[8]

Other important legal rights that were developed in the 1970s included federal regulations regarding the protection of research subjects and state laws and court decisions protecting medical privacy and confidentiality and

granting patients access to their medical records. The basic right to emergency care was also protected. Proposals for the development of patient
rights advocates and ombudspersons were not adopted, however, and
patients were generally left on their own to attempt to exercise their rights.
Patients generally had recourse to the courts only after their rights had been
violated and they had been harmed.

Patient Rights in Managed Care

The key to understanding patient rights in managed care is to understand
managed care's attempt to transform the patient into a consumer. Individuals
can be considered consumers of health plans (if they have a choice of plan)
because they can make a choice based on cost and coverage. But usually
this choice is made by their employers, and even when it is not, it is much
more often based on cost than on knowledge of coverage or quality. In
virtually all settings, *patients* (not consumers) seek the help of physicians
when they are sick and vulnerable because of illness or disability. The courts
in the 1970s were correct: the doctor–patient relationship is not an arms-
length commercial or business transaction, it is a relationship in which trust
is essential—in which sick people, who are "not themselves" and who know
little about medicine, *must* trust their physicians to be on their side against
their pain, suffering, disease, and disability.

Attempts to transform the doctor–patient relationship into a business
transaction fundamentally threaten not just physicians as professionals, but
people as patients. This threat remains real, frightening, and intolerable. This
is why the new patient rights movement is aimed not only at trying to protect the physician–patient relationship in general, but more specifically at neu-
tralizing the financial conflicts of interest in managed care that are most
threatening to it.[9] The new patient rights movement seeks not to shift power
from physicians and hospitals to patients, but from managed care companies, insurance companies, and health care facilities to patients *and* their
physicians.

Some threats featured in the media have been the subject of federal
legislation. Perhaps the most familiar was the "drive-through delivery" phe-
nomenon. Congress and a majority of states responded to managed care's
limitation on hospital stays following childbirth by mandating a minimal
stay when physician and patient agree that it is needed. The core response
to a perception that health plans had gone too far was predictable: an attempt to return decision-making power to a consensual and informed doctor–patient relationship freed from financial conflicts of interest.[10]

In 1997 in response to proposals to limit "drive-through mastectomies" (modeled after the drive-through delivery legislation), the American Association of Health Plans (AAHP) offered its "Putting Patients First" plan, also known as the "Nine Commandments."[11] This plan was almost immediately characterized by the editor of *The New England Journal of Medicine* as "a thinly veiled attempt to ward off state and federal legislative actions to curb the abuses of managed care," and it may have been.[12] Nonetheless, the content is instructive. None of the provisions of the nine commandments reproduce earlier patient bills of rights. Rather, they all have to do with areas in which health plans have been widely criticized for seeming to go too far, or concern areas in which medical decisions are being made by nonphysicians. For example, AAHP's proposal informs members (not patients or consumers) how the health plan works (how utilization review is done, drug formularies are set up, doctors are paid, and treatments are designated experimental); puts hospitalization for mastectomy treatment in the hands of physicians and their patients; removes any "gag rules" restricting physician conversations with patients about treatment options; describes appeals rights; and promises "physician involvement" in quality improvement programs, practice guidelines, and drug formulary development.

The AAHP proposal is similar in spirit to the National Commission on Quality Assurance's (NCQA) statement of "Members Rights and Responsibilities," which primarily focuses on informing members of health plans about their contract with the plan, especially the rules the health plan has adopted to make benefit coverage decisions, and how the plan will resolve complaints and disputes. These documents do not qualify as patient rights statements in any meaningful way because they concentrate only on contractual provisions.

The 18 "Principles for Consumer Protection" promoted by Kaiser, HIP, AARP, and Families USA seemed to go one step further, but it was a small and pathetic step. Other than those that duplicate provisions in the AAHP and NCQA documents, the essence of the recommendations is to require all health plans to provide certain services (such as out-of-area emergency coverage; 24-hour-a-day, 7-day-a-week medical services; and continuity of care through a primary care physician), disclose specific information (such as loss ratio), and restrict financial incentives that create physician–patient conflicts of interest (such as not encouraging provider groups to limit medically necessary care by financial incentives). As the authors concede, these 18 points are meant not primarily to help patients or customers, but as a marketing strategy to help these health plans compete against other health plans on a more equal basis.[13]

The basic weakness and almost irrelevance of these consumer–contract proposals to the typical patient makes much more comprehensive federal legislation on patient rights seem both necessary and desirable. Federal law is also the only way to protect all patients (in or out of health plans) and the only way to level the playing field for all health plans in the United States. What rights provisions should be included in national legislation?

The Presidential Commission

In early 1997 President Bill Clinton took the first step toward a National Patient Bill of Rights by appointing a Presidential Advisory Commission on Consumer Protection and Quality in the Health Care Industry (PAC). In late 1997 the PAC issued its proposal. Although flawed and incomplete, it nonetheless provided a basic outline for a national patient bill of rights.[14] PAC divides its major areas of concern into what may be described as four fundamental post-1970 patient rights (informed choice, confidentiality, emergency care, and respect), and three contract-based consumer rights (contract information, choice of physician within a plan, and access to an independent appeals mechanism).

The core of patient rights (which should also be the core of medical ethics) is the right to receive care from an accountable physician who shares all relevant information with the patient and guarantees the patient the right to make the final decision. The patient must be able to trust the physician to act honestly and in the patient's best interests. Loyalty to the patient also requires the physician to act as an advocate for the patient when the treatment the physician believes is most appropriate for the patient is not covered by the patient's health plan or insurance. Only provisions that honor and reinforce a mutual physician–patient relationship worthy of trust deserve to be designated patient rights.

Consumer protection is also important but pales in comparison to what sick people need from their physicians. Thus, the PAC is directly on target to stipulate that any bill of patient rights include the following: a right to complete treatment information, a right to emergency care based on what a prudent layperson would regard as an emergency, a right to privacy of medical information, and a right to respectful and nondiscriminatory treatment. As for managed care rights, it is pretty thin gruel to guarantee members access to the contract they or their employer signed. Nonetheless, the call for an external, independent grievance mechanism for benefit denials was welcome (and needed) because the internal grievance mechanisms available to patients were woefully inadequate in virtually all health plans.[15] The PAC should have gone further. Patients need access to an effective patient rights advocate to help them exercise all the rights spelled out in any bill of patient rights. An advocate could also help them, together with their physician, navigate the grievance and appeals mechanisms with the goal of resolving disputes at the lowest possible level and as quickly and fairly as possible.[16]

A National Patient Bill of Rights

The final shape of a national bill of patient rights has been debated in Congress on and off through mid-2004 without resolution. The model adopted, whether consumer–contract or physician–patient oriented, and whether implemented voluntarily or by federal legislation will largely determine the ultimate content. And the ultimate content will also determine whether federal preemption of this area is reasonable. We can call people who purchase health insurance consumers, and people who join health plans can be called members. However, we must recognize (and protect through enforceable rights) that sick people who seek medical care are patients. A national bill of patient rights can and should protect consumers and members of managed care plans. But its core purpose must be to provide all Americans with basic rights at the time it means most to all of us: when we are sick and need medical care.

Many of our rights as patients have already been articulated by the courts. Nonetheless, they often remain difficult for patients and providers alike to understand and especially difficult for sick people to exercise.[17] Thus, it is helpful to collect all major patient rights in one document for both educational and enforcement ease and to provide an effective and fair mechanism to permit patients to actually exercise their rights in the real world, with their physicians and hospitals. To be constructive I believe a national bill of patient rights must include at least the following five core elements.

Treatment Information

The patient has a right to informed participation in all decisions involving the patient's health care, including a clear, concise explanation, in laypersons' terms, of all proposed procedures, the reasonable medical alternatives, the risks of death and serious complications of each (including no treatment), likely problems of recuperation, and the probability of success (including the physician's experience with the treatment and outcomes the physician has had with it). The patient has a right to know the diagnosis and prognosis in as much detail as desired, as well as the existence of any research protocols that are relevant to the patient's condition and their availability. The patient will not be subjected to any procedures or tests without voluntary, competent, and understanding consent. For procedures that entail a risk of death or serious disability, all aspects of informed consent will be set out in a written form requiring the signature of the patient or the individual with authority to make treatment decisions for the patient if the patient is incompetent.

The patient has a right to know the identity of the primary physician as well as the identity, professional status, experience, and clinical outcomes of all persons responsible for his or her care. The patient has a right to know of all financial arrangements and incentives that might affect his or her care.

The Right to Privacy and Dignity

The patient has a right to privacy of both person and information with respect to all medical, nursing, allied health, health plan, and facility staff members and other patients. All patients must be treated with dignity and without regard to race, religion, sex, sexual orientation, national origin, disability, age, socioeconomic status, or source of payment. The patient has a right to all the information contained in his or her medical record and has a right to examine the record on request, correct mistakes, and receive a copy of it. No one not directly involved in a patient's care or in quality assurance should have access to the patient's medical records without a written authorization by the patient that is dated and limited in time and that specifies the medical information to be disclosed. Further disclosure of medical information without authorization is prohibited. The patient has a right not to be touched or treated by any particular physician or health care provider, including medical and nursing students.

The Right to Refuse Treatment

The patient has the right to refuse any intervention, including a drug, test, procedure, or treatment, whether for therapy, research, or education. Patients may not be discriminated against or denied any benefit from a health plan or health professional because of a refusal. A patient has the right to execute a health care proxy or a living will to direct treatment or nontreatment when the patient is no longer capable of making health care decisions, and health care professionals are obligated to comply with these advance directives.

The Right to Emergency Care

The patient has a right to prompt and competent attention in an emergency, including the right to a clear, complete, and accurate evaluation of the patient's condition and prognosis before being asked to consent to any test or procedure. The patient may not be transferred to another facility without the patient's consent, and in any event, not before the patient has been stabilized and it has been determined that transfer is in the patient's best interests because of superior medical care at the other facility. If the patient does not agree to transfer, the patient may not be transferred.

The Right to an Advocate

The patient has the right to the services of an independent patient rights advocate with the authority to help the patient assert all the rights specified in the bill of rights. This advocate will usually be a friend or family member. In addition, a patient in a hospital or other health care facility has the right to reasonable visitation, parents have the right to stay with their child, and relatives have the right to stay with patients 24 hours a day. The patient has the right to have a friend or relative, or other advocate present during all consultations, examinations, and procedures, including the induction of anesthesia.

Other Provisions

Additional provisions of a national patient bill of rights will involve contract-based consumer protections.[18] How specifically such provisions will be spelled out will depend on the extent to which Congress believes health plan contracts must be regulated. In any event, the following obligations of health plans should be included. No health plan may interfere with or limit communication between the patient and his or her health care provider. Health plans must provide members with a reasonable choice of qualified primary care physicians and reasonable access to specialists. Health plans must disclose to members any and all financial arrangements that might encourage physicians to limit or restrict care, referrals to specialists, or recommendations of noncovered treatments. Health plans must provide payment for emergency services under circumstances that a prudent layperson would consider an emergency. Health plans must provide timely access to an independent appeals mechanism for denial or termination of benefits. The patient has a right to a copy of the entire contract for his or her insurance or health plan and to competent counseling in selecting a health plan. The patient has a right, regardless of the source of payment, to examine and receive an itemized and detailed explanation of all services rendered. The patient has a right to timely prior notice of termination of eligibility for coverage or denial of a health care benefit, with an opportunity to contest the termination or denial in a timely and fair manner before an independent, qualified, and neutral decision maker.

A national bill of patient rights must cover all Americans. On the other hand, health plans must be held accountable for providing the health and medical care to their members that they hold themselves out as being able to provide. Thus, Congress should also pass legislation that permits injured patient-members to sue their health plans directly for harm caused by their wrongful acts.

Once basic, uniform rights in health care are established, we can return to the urgent task of providing access to health care for all Americans. It seems correct to view universal access to decent health care as our primary goal. But rights in health care are critical, since without them citizens may wind up with access to a system that is indifferent to both their suffering and their rights. Medical ethics in particular, and bioethics in general, have simply been unable (or unwilling) to protect the basic human rights of patients. This is why health law is necessary, and, because its principles are enforceable in court, why American bioethics has not only followed health law, but, in the context of the doctor–patient relationship, has been eclipsed by health law.

Rights and rights talk nonetheless remain foreign to many physicians. Perhaps because of the great deference courts usually show physicians in complicated cases (such as the separation of conjoined twins), some physicians seem to believe that they can follow their own ethical compass without regard to the law—at least in what they see as life-and-death cases. The next chapter explores cases in which physicians have acted lawlessly and have had to be reminded that the law, not their idiosyncratic view of medical ethics, really does govern their actions.

9

. . . .

White Coat Police

T he supreme value in America is liberty, and this is reflected not only in American law, but in American bioethics as well, usually under the rubric of autonomy. Informed consent is the doctrine designed to ensure that patients understand what is proposed to be done to them so they can make an informed choice to accept or reject it. The practice of medicine is, in short, a voluntary activity between two consenting adults. But in rare instances some physicians have forgotten this underlying principle of the doctor–patient relationship and acted more like police officers dealing with a criminal suspect. When physicians act like police, they can become even more arbitrary and abusive than actual police because they justify their actions not for the good of society, but for the good of their patient. Such justification can lead to ghoulish coercion. This chapter details two contrasting examples, one from the emergency department of a private teaching hospital with no direct police involvement, the other from the outpatient clinic of a public hospital that was working directly with the police.[1]

Restraints in the Emergency Department

Catherine Shine, the 29-year-old daughter of a physician, suffered a severe asthma attack on a Sunday morning in March 1990 while at her sister Anna's apartment. Catherine had asthma most of her life, and was well informed about her illness. Her attacks were characterized by a rapid onset and rapid remission. She controlled her asthma with medication and had never required intubation.[2]

Anna suggested that they go to Massachusetts General Hospital. Catherine agreed, but only if her treatment would be limited to the administration of oxygen. Anna called the hospital and was assured that Catherine would be treated only with oxygen. They went to the emergency department at 7 A.M., where Catherine was given oxygen and medication through a nebulizer. Catherine soon removed the nebulizer, reporting that the medication gave her a headache, and said she wanted to leave the hospital. This behavior alarmed the treating nurse. Blood gas results, obtained at about 7:30 A.M., showed that she was "very sick." José Vega, the only attending physician on duty in the emergency department that morning, examined Catherine and concluded that intubation was necessary. Catherine refused, and Vega agreed to continue treatment with the oxygen mask. Anna meanwhile telephoned their physician father, Ian Shine, in England. Shine spoke with the physician and told him that Catherine understood her illness well and that he should listen to her and not treat her without her consent. Vega testified that he told Shine that he had to intubate Catherine because she was "in the midst of a severe asthma attack" and that Shine asked him to wait until he flew to Boston before attempting the intubation.

When Anna returned to Catherine's room, her sister's condition had improved somewhat. Catherine was able to talk and breathe more easily, but she was in a heated argument with the staff. At about 7:40 A.M., when they were left alone for a moment, Catherine told Anna to "run"; they ran down the corridor to an exit door, where they were forcibly apprehended by a physician and a security guard. Catherine was returned to her room, and Vega immediately ordered her placed in four-point restraints. Anna was removed from the room and not allowed to speak with her sister or observe her treatment. At approximately 8 A.M., new blood gas results indicated that Catherine's condition had improved; Vega did not read the new test results and testified that they would not have affected his decision to intubate her in any case.

At approximately 8:25 A.M. Catherine was forcibly intubated. She had been in four-point restraints for about 45 minutes. No one ever questioned

Catherine's competence to consent to treatment, nor was there any basis on which to question her competence. Catherine never consented to intubation, and Vega testified that he never discussed the risks and benefits of intubation with Catherine, Anna, or their father. Catherine's condition subsequently improved, and she was released from the hospital the following day.

Catherine was severely traumatized by her mistreatment at the hospital. She had nightmares, cried constantly, was unable to return to work for several months, became obsessed about her medication, and swore repeatedly that she would never go to a hospital again. Approximately two years later Catherine had a severe asthma attack while at home with her fiance and her brother. She refused to be taken to a hospital. Her brother, nonetheless, called an ambulance after she became unconscious, which transported her to a nearby hospital. After unsuccessful medical treatment, she died.

Her father, as administrator of her estate, brought a multicount lawsuit against Vega and Massachusetts General Hospital, alleging, among other things, negligence, assault and battery, false imprisonment, and wrongful death. Her father's primary contention, both at the trial and on appeal, was that Vega wrongfully restrained and intubated Catherine without her consent. Vega and the hospital took the position that because Catherine was suffering a life-threatening emergency, consent was not necessary. The trial judge instructed the jury that "under Massachusetts law a patient has the right to refuse medical treatment except in an emergency, life-threatening situation." The jury returned a verdict in favor of the defendants on all counts. Catherine's father appealed. The Supreme Judicial Court took the case directly, and all seven justices, in a unanimous decision, found that the jury instructions were erroneous, vacated the judgment, and remanded the case for a new trial.

The Law of Physical Restraints

The opinion, written by Chief Justice Margaret Marshall, held that both common law and constitutional law provide for the "right of a competent individual to refuse medical treatment." The court had ruled in a previous case that the "right to bodily integrity" had developed through the doctrine of informed consent, under which "a physician has the duty to disclose to a competent adult sufficient information to enable the patient to make an informed judgment whether to give or withhold consent to a medical or surgical procedure." The patient's decision need not be a "wise" one, and the right to refuse treatment includes the right to refuse "life-saving procedures."[3]

This restates well-established law, although the fact that the trial court judge did not know the law is disturbing. Appeals courts, however, exist to correct such errors. The defendants had argued that there is an exception to the informed consent doctrine in the case of lifesaving treatment rendered in an emergency department, which includes the use of restraints as part of treatment. The court was sympathetic to the emergency department physicians but ruled that the need for quick action in an emergency cannot justify ignorance of the law or indifference to basic legal rights. In the words of the court:

> If the patient is competent, an emergency physician must obtain her consent before providing treatment, even if the physician is persuaded that, without the treatment, the patient's life is threatened. If the patient's consent cannot be obtained because the patient is unconscious or otherwise incapable of consenting, the emergency physician should seek the consent of a family member if time and circumstances permit.

The court also quoted a standard law textbook that summarizes the three basic requirements for emergency treatment without consent:

> (a) The patient must be unconscious or without capacity to make a decision, while no one legally authorized to act as agent for the patient is available; (b) time must be of the essence, in the sense that it must reasonably appear that delay until such time as an effective consent could be obtained would subject the patient to a risk of serious bodily injury or death which prompt action would avoid; and (c) under the circumstances, a reasonable person would consent, and the probabilities are that the patient would consent.[4]

The defendants did not contend that Catherine was incompetent (i.e., not able to understand and appreciate the nature and consequences of her decisions) but rather that after she was prevented from leaving the hospital, she "became more confused and combative, refusing treatment." Her responses, however, were reasonable rejoinders to the physician's actions and not evidence of incompetence. An assessment of competence in this case would have required Catherine to answer only two questions: Did she know what the physician wanted to do and why? And did she know that she could die if the intervention were not performed?[5] The answer to both these questions was indisputably yes. Of course, even had it been determined that Catherine was incompetent, her sister and father would have had the authority to make decisions on her behalf consistent with her directions, not her physician.

Federal regulations adopted after this case prohibit the use of restraints as a means of coercion—the way they were used to prevent Catherine from leaving the hospital. The standard for restraint for acute medical and surgical care is:

> (1) The patient has the right to be free from restraints of any form that are not medically necessary or are used as a means of coercion, discipline, convenience, or retaliation by staff. . . . (2) A restraint can only be used if needed to improve the patient's well-being and less restrictive interventions have been determined to be ineffective. . . . (3) The use of restraint must be . . . in accordance with the order of a physician or other licensed independent practitioner [and] . . . never written as a standing [or as needed] order. . . . (4) The condition of the restrained patient must be continually assessed, monitored, and reevaluated.

There is a separate standard for the use of seclusion and restraints for behavior management. (Seclusion is not allowed at all under the standard for medical care.) This standard resembles the medical and surgical standard but is stricter, including provisions that "seclusion or restraint can only be used in emergency situations if needed to ensure the patient's physical safety and less restrictive interventions have been determined to be ineffective," that a "physician or other licensed independent practitioner must see [the patient] and evaluate the need for restraint or seclusion within 1 hour after the initiation of this intervention," and that orders must be written and must be "limited to [a period of] 4 hours for adults; 2 hours for children and adolescents ages 9 to 17 or 1 hour for patients under 9." Once the original order expires, a physician must see and assess the patient before a new order can be issued. Physical restraints include both mechanical devices and drugs used to "control behavior or to restrict the patient's freedom of movement." Unfortunately, the rules do not make it clear enough that behavior management is only to prevent a patient from harming himself or herself (such as by hitting his or her head against a wall or attempting suicide) or from harming others. Behavior management to avoid harm to others is closer to a policing function than to treatment. Because they require a physician's order, the patient's primary protection against the use of restraints under the regulations is reliance on medical ethics through the requirement of a physician's order. But this, of course, offers no protection at all in a case in which the physician believes medical ethics supports, or even requires, the use of restraints.

Two other provisions in the regulations might have helped Catherine. Four-point restraints are almost never the least restrictive means available, and the regulations require that the use of a restraint must be "selected only when other less restrictive measures have been found to be ineffective to protect the patient or others from harm." Following this rule would have required at a minimum a rational explanation, followed by the use of verbal threats and a show of physical intimidation (neither of which would have been acceptable in this case, but both of which would have been "less restrictive") before the actual use of physical restraints. The regulations also require that the use of restraints be "ended at the earliest possible time." After Catherine's second blood gas test showed that her condition was improving, neither treatment nor restraint was necessary. The blood gas levels were not rechecked by the physician, but if the regulations had been in effect, such a reassessment would have been required because the regulations state that "the condition of the restrained patient must be continually assessed, monitored, and reevaluated."[6]

As originally proposed, the rules included the phrase that restraints could be "used only as a last resort." A number of commentators suggested that this phrase be replaced with "when medically necessary." As the Massachusetts case illustrates, however, this phrase can make the decision to use restraints seem like a medical one and substitutes personal medical ethics for law. Catherine's physician might have thought, for example, that his use of restraints was "medically necessary." The federal agency decided against the use of either phrase and instead replaced "as a last resort" with the phrase "when other less restrictive measures have been found to be ineffective."[7] I think this was a mistake. The agency was right not to see the use of restraints as a standard medical procedure, but the agency was wrong to back down. The overall point of the regulations is that restraints and seclusion are to be used only if absolutely necessary, and the language that best expresses this and alerts all staff members that the use of restraints should be extremely unusual is that they should be used "only as a last resort."

The only justification for the use of restraints in an emergency is to prevent patients from physically harming themselves (if the patient is not competent) or others, and even then they should be used only for the shortest time possible and with the least restriction possible. Competent adult patients retain the right to refuse treatment, even in the emergency setting. Coercive measures, including restraints and the threat of restraints, cannot be justifiably used simply because a patient refuses treatment because this would destroy the very value informed consent is designed to protect: the right of choice.

Neither health law nor the federal regulations permit the use of restraints in Catherine Shine's case. It is, moreover, almost always the case in disputes between a physician and a competent patient over a recommended treatment that the most effective approach is to continue to discuss with the patient the reasons for the recommendation, the alternatives, and the consequences of doing nothing. This approach takes time, but even in an emergency there is no substitute. The patient's family is often useful in this situation, not because the family has any legal authority to consent on behalf of a competent patient, but because family members might help the physician understand the patient and might also help the patient understand the physician.

It can also be very useful to contact the patient's primary care physician. Facts can be ascertained, especially about past treatment. Physical assessment, however, may not be possible. Neither the person at Massachusetts General Hospital who assured Anna that Catherine would get only oxygen nor her physician father, who was in England, could properly assess Catherine's condition over the telephone. This is why the federal regulations properly insist on the actual presence of a physician. Continued discussion is important because a patient who understands the recommended intervention and its rationale is much more likely to agree to it. A refusal under these circumstances is more likely to be an informed one as well, and treatment refusals as well as treatment acceptances must be informed.[8] Competent patients, however, cannot be forced either to talk or to listen, and the fact that they will not talk to their physician does not by itself make them incompetent.

Catherine Shine, as a competent adult patient, also had a legal right to leave the hospital at any time she decided to leave. Hospitals are not prisons, and patients do not check their legal rights at the door when they enter. Catherine should have been allowed to leave the hospital because she was competent. In contrast, when Catherine's brother and fiance accompanied her to another emergency department when she was unconscious, the physicians there could (and did) properly treat her on the authorization of these persons. The only time emergency department physicians should not treat an unconscious patient is if the physicians know that the patient would not accept a particular treatment, even if it was thought to be necessary to prevent death. This raises difficult issues of proof, but if Catherine either had had a prior relationship with the physician during which this had been discussed, or had completed an advance directive forbidding intubation under such circumstances, then her directive would have been legally decisive, regardless of the wishes of her family.

The overarching general rule is that informed consent is required before physicians can lawfully treat competent adult patients, all of whom have the right to refuse medical treatment. Patients who consent to interventions such as surgery, of course, agree to the reasonable use of drugs and physical restraints during surgery and postoperatively while they are disoriented. But in most other circumstances, few competent patients would agree to be restrained. Insofar as they continue the move away from medical paternalism toward the protection of patients and their rights, the federal restraint regulations are to be applauded. However, the absence of a clear statement that they apply only to incompetent patients leaves the regulations open to potentially dangerous misinterpretation. And to the extent that they make the use of restraints seem legitimate and medically appropriate in some settings, they fall short of conveying the message that restraints should be used only as a last resort. Physicians may be even more disposed to use coercion if they believe they are furthering important public health goals, such as trying to prevent premature births.

Physicians as Drug Law Enforcers

In 1989 Supreme Court Justice Thurgood Marshall surmised that "declaring a war on illegal drugs is good public policy . . . [but] the first, and worst, casualty of war will be the precious liberties of our citizens."[9] The same year, in the midst of President George Bush's "war on drugs," the Medical University of South Carolina initiated a program to screen selected pregnant patients for cocaine and to provide positive test results to the police.[10] At a time of high public concern about "cocaine babies," university and local public officials adopted this policy. Drug screening programs in other groups of people had been found constitutional by the Supreme Court, and it was beginning to appear that the war on drugs would claim the Fourth Amendment, which prohibits unreasonable searches, as one of its first casualties.[11] In 2001, however, the Supreme Court found the university's policy constitutionally deficient.[12]

The university policy, developed with the local police department, ultimately provided that a pregnant woman who tested positive for cocaine would be given a letter from the local prosecutor saying that if she successfully completed a drug treatment program she would not be prosecuted. If she did not complete the program, however, the police would be notified and she would be arrested and charged with simple drug possession if her pregnancy was 27 weeks or less, possession and drug distribution if 28 weeks or more. If she tested positive at the time of delivery, she would also be charged with child neglect. Pregnant women were to be tested for cocaine if they met any of nine criteria: the receipt of no prenatal care, of late prenatal care after 24 weeks' gestation, or of incomplete prenatal care; abruptio placentae; intrauterine fetal death; preterm labor "of no obvious cause"; intrauterine growth retardation "of no obvious cause"; previously known drug or alcohol abuse; and unexplained congenital anomalies. Although he helped initiate the program, the hospital's general counsel worried about the hospital's potential liability. For example, he wrote to the state's attorney general that he would "prefer to have the mothers sign an informed consent to the drug screen [and that] the DSS [Department of Social Services] be notified rather than law enforcement. . . ."[13]

Under the policy, which was in effect until 1994, 253 women tested positive for cocaine. Thirty of them were arrested, and two were sentenced to prison. Ten of the women who were arrested sued for violation of their constitutional rights. They were represented by the American Civil Liberties Union. Of the 10, 9 were black. All were poor. Six had been arrested at the hospital shortly after giving birth. Three had been arrested when they failed to complete a drug treatment program. The only white woman of the 10 was told at a prenatal visit that she must either voluntarily admit herself to a psychiatric unit or be arrested. She spent 30 days in the unit before giving birth. The lawsuit was filed in 1993.

The university discontinued its policy in 1994 in a settlement agreement with the Civil Rights Division of the U.S. Department of Health and Human Services, which was investigating whether the policy violated the Civil Rights Act. In that same month, the Office for Protection from Research Risks of the National Institutes of Health, after investigating a complaint, notified the university that its cocaine testing policy constituted a research project that had not been reviewed by the institutional review board, a violation of federal regulations.

Because the women were suing for monetary damages, and because the university would not agree to discontinue using noncriminal coercive measures, including civil commitment, their lawsuit against the university, the city, and the police continued even though the arrest policy had been abandoned. The Fourth Amendment provides that "the right of the people to be secure in their persons, houses, papers, and effects, against unreasonable search and seizures, shall not be violated, and no Warrants shall issue, but upon probable cause, supported by Oath or affirmation, and particularly describing the place to be searched, and the person or things to be seized." The amendment prohibits unreasonable searches by the police or those working for the police without a warrant or the consent of the person searched, unless there is some "special non-law-enforcement need" for the search that makes it reasonable. At the trial, the defendants offered two defenses for testing the urine of the pregnant women for cocaine: first, the women had in fact consented to the searches, so no warrant was necessary; and second, even without consent, the searches were justified by a "special non-law-enforcement need." The trial court rejected the second defense but put the first one to the jury, instructing the jury that it had to find in favor of the women unless it found they had consented to the search. The jury found in favor of the defendants. The women appealed.

The Fourth Circuit Court of Appeals affirmed the verdict in a two-to-one opinion.[14] The circuit court held that the searches were reasonable under the Fourth Amendment as a matter of law because of the "special need" to protect women and children from the complications of the maternal use of cocaine. The dissenting judge disagreed and also concluded that the evidence of consent was insufficient to sustain the jury's verdict. The women appealed to the U.S. Supreme Court.

In a six-to-three opinion, the Supreme Court reversed the decision of the circuit court regarding the special needs exception and sent the case back to the circuit court for a factual determination of whether the women had actually consented to the searches. Justice John Paul Stevens wrote the opinion of the Court, focusing on the special needs exception. That exception had been adopted in 1989 by the Supreme Court in two cases. One involved testing railway workers for drugs and alcohol after major train accidents. The other involved testing U.S. Customs employees for drug use when they were seeking sensitive jobs or promotions. The special needs exception had also been used to justify the drug testing of high school students participating in interscholastic sports.[15] It had, however, been found insufficient to make drug testing a condition for filing candidate papers for certain state offices.[16]

Justice Stevens concluded that in each of these cases the Court had used a "balancing test that weighed the intrusion on the individual's interest in privacy against the 'special needs' that supported the program." The purpose of testing railway workers, for example, was to try to learn the cause of accidents so as to prevent them; the Customs employees were tested to make sure they could not easily be compromised by drug smugglers; high school athletes were tested to see whether they were eligible for an extracurricular activity. Stevens observed that the non-law-enforcement purpose of the drug tests in all these special needs cases was clear and that precautions were taken to ensure that the police did not obtain the results.

Justice Stevens found that the "critical difference" between the previous special needs cases and this one was the "nature of the 'special need' asserted for the warrantless search." Specifically, Stevens concluded that whereas the special need in each of the previous cases was "divorced from the State's general interest in law enforcement," in South Carolina "the central and indispensable feature of the [drug testing] policy from its inception was the use of law enforcement to coerce the patients into substance abuse treatment."

The drug testing policy of the Medical University of South Carolina, Stevens concluded, was "ultimately indistinguishable from the [state's] general interest in crime control." This conclusion followed from the fact that the police helped to develop the program, were involved in its day-to-day administration, determined the procedures to be followed, and coordinated the "timing and circumstances of the arrests with [university] staff," and that women were jailed. In Justice Stevens's words, "The threat of law enforcement may ultimately have been intended as the means to an end, but the direct and primary purpose of [the university's] policy was to ensure the use of those means. In our opinion, this distinction is critical."

The Court sent the question of whether the women had consented back to the circuit court for further consideration. According to the trial judge's instructions to the jury, in order to find that the women had provided informed consent, the jury had to conclude not only that the women consented to have a urine sample taken for medical testing but also that they consented to have their urine tested for cocaine knowing that the results of the testing would be turned over to the police. Even though the jury did find that consent had been provided, the dissenting judge in the Fourth Circuit Court decision believed that there was insufficient evidence for them to reach this conclusion. The consent form that was used, for example, was general and vague, providing simply that "attending physicians, members of the House Staff, and the Medical University Clinics have my permission to reveal information to appropriate agencies and individuals where it becomes necessary to protect the welfare of myself/the patient and/ or the community." Far from being evidence that informed consent to share incriminating evidence of drug use with the police was obtained, the form is evidence that it was not. Nothing in the form indicated to the patient that her consent could lead to arrest and imprisonment.

When the case was remanded by the Supreme Court, the Court of Appeals ruled that in order to give their informed consent the women had to know that "the primary purpose of the urine drug screens was crime detection, not medical treatment." Moreover, they had to be able to refuse it without negative consequences. The court reviewed the facts of each case

and concluded that the evidence presented at trial was insufficient for any
rational jury to find that any of the defendants consented to the drug testing. The court therefore returned the case to the trial court for a determination of damages involving all of the defendants except one (who was not
tested, but whose baby's urine was tested for cocaine).[17]

The Role of Physicians

Justice Anthony Kennedy wrote a concurring opinion arguing that cocaine
use during pregnancy is terrible and that the state has the authority to oppose
and punish it, although he agreed that the Fourth Amendment limits what
the state can do. In his words, the state is legitimately concerned with "the
grave risk to the life and health of the fetus, and later the child, caused by
cocaine ingestion . . . South Carolina can impose punishment upon an
expectant mother who has so little regard for her own unborn that she risks
causing him or her lifelong damage and suffering."

Justice Antonin Scalia wrote a dissenting opinion for himself, Chief
Justice William Rehnquist and Justice Clarence Thomas, which is most
notable for its peculiar view of physicians and the doctor–patient relationship. Scalia believes that as long as a pregnant woman consents to having
her urine taken, it is irrelevant whether she knows what it will be tested for
or who will obtain the test results. He remarkably compared the relationship between a doctor and a patient to that between a suspected criminal
and a police informant who has gained the confidence of a suspect. Information voluntarily disclosed by the suspect to the police informant can be
used against the suspect. Scalia thinks the same principle should apply to
patients. In his words, "information obtained through violation of a relationship of trust is obtained consensually, and is hence not a search."

Even if this conclusion is rejected, Scalia argued, the special needs
exception should still apply: there is no difference, argued Scalia, between
the actions of the physicians in this case and their actions in adherence to
specific statutes that require them to report certain findings, such as gunshot wounds, to the police. Scalia compared physicians to probation officers (and patients to convicted criminals), seeing no difference between a
probation officer's search of a parolee's home for a gun and the physician's
search of a patient's body for cocaine. He concluded with his view that the
primary purpose of the policy at the Medical University of South Carolina
was not law enforcement but the provision of health benefits to the women
through the identification of a "drug-impaired mother and child for necessary medical treatment."

For more than a decade, it seemed that the war on drugs in the United States would gut the Fourth Amendment.[18] The trend toward approving searches of urine for the presence of drugs, however, has now been stalled, if not stopped. The reasonable expectation of privacy in the doctor–patient relationship renders unreasonable under the Fourth Amendment nonconsensual searches for the presence of illegal drugs as part of a plan to turn this information over to the police. As the majority of the Court stressed, it is one thing to require physicians to report certain findings from the ordinary course of administering treatment, such as evidence of child abuse or neglect or even gunshot wounds. It is another thing for physicians to work directly with the police to search for evidence of criminal behavior. In the first instance, the physician practices medicine and only performs tests and procedures that are medically indicated for the care of the patient. In the second instance, the physician becomes an agent of the police, conducting a criminal investigation that is outside the domain of medicine and certainly not expected by patients.

There is, nonetheless, some tension inherent in mandatory reporting laws that the Court does not acknowledge. Reporting statutes that are aimed at preventing harm to children, such as the reporting of child abuse and neglect to state agencies charged with protecting children, can be seen as consistent with the physician's obligation to the child. No parent has (or should have) the reasonable expectation that a physician will keep evidence of child abuse or neglect from the state's child protection agency, because both the physician and the state have obligations to act in the best interests of children by protecting them from serious harm. Moreover, the child protection agency is not a police or law enforcement agency; its only function is to protect the welfare of children by providing protective services to them.

Mandatory reporting of gunshot wounds and knife wounds, however, is more difficult to reconcile with the duties of physicians, which should be to care for the wounded person (who can report the source of the wound to the authorities himself or herself) rather than assisting the police to identify the assailant. Such reporting can, however, be seen as protective of the patient insofar as it triggers a police hunt for the assailant, and this goal is consistent with the patient's interests. Moreover, the patient is not being accused of a crime. Nonetheless, as the Court recognized, the more physicians and nurses become entangled in law enforcement, the more they resemble agents of the police (and police informants and probation officers) rather than health care professionals. Physicians' role in law enforcement, in turn, undermines the trust patients place in them and thus the very ability of physicians to practice medicine; distrustful patients will not be candid with physicians and may even avoid them altogether.[19] During pregnancy, the avoidance of prenatal care can be more devastating to the fetus than drug use.

Medical research fails to support the contention that the exposure of a fetus to cocaine is uniquely harmful. Rather, the evidence supports the hypothesis that cocaine exposure is itself correlated with other harmful factors, including poverty, malnutrition, and exposure to tobacco, marijuana, and alcohol.[20] Thus, there is no medical justification for a special intervention related only to fetal exposure to cocaine. Nonetheless, Justice Kennedy supports state laws that criminalize behaviors during pregnancy that he believes harm the fetus (and thus the child), and that treat pregnant women more severely than others who commit the same crime. He sees punishing the mother after the birth of the child as appropriate, although it is difficult to see how putting a new mother in jail helps her newborn baby or her other children.

In coming to his conclusion, Kennedy ignores the reasoning behind the decision of the Court in the 1991 case of *Johnson Controls*.[21] In that case, the question was whether a private employer could, consistent with Title VII of the Civil Rights Act of 1964 and the Pregnancy Discrimination Act of 1978, exclude women who could become pregnant from working in jobs that exposed them to lead because such exposure could harm fetuses. The Court found that being infertile is not "a bona fide occupational qualification" for making batteries. Put another way, employers cannot convert a general desire to protect the health of fetuses into a job qualification, because this would exclude almost all women from any job that might have a negative impact on fetuses. In the Court's words, "women as capable of doing their job as their male counterparts may not be forced to choose between having a child and having a job." Although Kennedy agreed with the holding in that case, he joined a concurring opinion of Justice Byron White that argued that under other circumstances it might be reasonable for an employer to consider the fetus a "third party" whose safety was, like that of its customers, its responsibility.

In *Johnson Controls*, the Court noted that Congress had left the welfare of the next generation to parents, not employers, and wrote that "Decisions about the welfare of future children must be left to the parents who conceive, bear, support, and raise them rather than to the employers who hire those parents." The same reasoning applies to drug abuse. Drug abuse is a major public health problem, as is exposure to lead, but to penalize pregnant women more than other women and men for the same act makes pregnancy itself the real crime. *Johnson Controls* was about interpreting a statute, whereas the South Carolina case involved an interpretation of the Constitution. Nonetheless, the rationale of fetal protection claimed by the supporters of the policies in both cases is the same. And in both cases, the Court concluded that the rights of women (whether statutory or constitutional) are not automatically forfeited because of pregnancy. Fetal protection cannot reasonably be used to justify uniquely restricting or criminalizing the activities of pregnant women.[22] This would start us down the slippery slope of controlling all behaviors of pregnant women, criminal or not, that might affect the health of their fetuses—not only alcohol use and smoking, but also working at certain jobs and engaging in some sports.[23]

Remarkably, Justice Thurgood Marshall's prediction that the war on drugs would spell the demise of the Fourth Amendment now appears far less likely to come true. A Court that strongly supports both law enforcement and the war on drugs has declared unequivocally that there are limits on the coercive tactics that can be used in that war, and some of these limits are set by the Fourth Amendment. The rights of pregnant women, however, remain severely contested, nowhere more so than in the area of so-called partial birth abortions, the subject of the next chapter, and as we will see, the legal rights of pregnant women are inextricably tied to the medical ethics of their physicians.

10

. . . .

Partial Birth Abortion

N o bioethics or health law issue in America has defied so many attempts to alter its contours as abortion.[1] Abortion was a contentious
issue in bioethics when American bioethics entered early ado-
lesence in the late 1960s, and it remains intransigent today. The political
and bioethics debates on abortion over the past 30 years have shifted among
various dichotomous views of the world: life versus choice, fetus versus
woman, fetus versus baby, constitutional rights versus state rights, government versus physician, and physician and patient versus state legislatures.
Hundreds of statutes and almost two dozen U.S. Supreme Court decisions
on abortion later, the essential aspects of *Roe v. Wade*,[2] the most controversial health-related Court decision in history, remain substantially the same
as they were in 1973. Both courtroom and legislative attempts to overturn
Roe have failed. Pregnant women have a constitutional right to choose
abortion. The fetus is not a person under the Constitution. States still cannot make abortion a crime (either for the woman or the physician) before
fetal viability. States can outlaw abortion after fetal viability only if there is
an exception that permits abortion to protect the life or health of the pregnant woman. And states can impose restrictions on abortion before fetal

viability only if those restrictions do not actually create a significant barrier to pregnant women who want to obtain an abortion.

The primary political tactic of the past decade has shifted from the use of antiabortion rhetoric to try to change the law concerning abortion to the use of legislative and judicial forums to change the rhetoric of abortion. The hope seems to be that more heated rhetoric, such as "partial birth abortion," will help turn the public and physicians against abortion itself, regardless of its constitutional protection.

Thirty years ago, in *Roe v. Wade*, the Supreme Court held that women have a constitutional right of privacy that is "fundamental" and "broad enough to encompass a woman's decision . . . to terminate her pregnancy." Because the right is fundamental, the state must demonstrate a compelling state interest to restrict it. The Court determined that the state's interest in the life of the fetus only became compelling at the point of viability, defined as when the fetus can survive independent of its mother. Moreover, the state cannot favor the life of the fetus over the life or health of the pregnant woman. In *Roe v. Wade* the Court held that even after a fetus is viable, physicians must be able to use their "medical judgment for the preservation of the life or health of the mother." *Roe*'s companion case, *Doe v. Bolton*, specifically included mental health in this determination, saying, "The medical judgment may be exercised in the light of all factors—physical, emotional, psychological, familial, and the woman's age—relevant to the well-being of the patient. All these factors may relate to health. This allows the attending physician the room he [*sic*] needs to make his best medical judgment."[3]

When the Court heard *Planned Parenthood v. Casey* in 1992, most commentators assumed that there were more than enough votes to overturn *Roe*.[4] Instead, three seemingly anti-*Roe* justices wrote a joint opinion confirming the "core holding" of *Roe*: that states could not outlaw abortion prior to fetal viability and could only do so thereafter when the life or health of the woman was not threatened by continuing the pregnancy. With the loss of all hope that the current Court would ever overturn *Roe*, antiabortion advocates needed a new approach to keep the abortion debate alive. They found it in the rare use of so-called partial birth abortion.

Partial Birth Abortion in Congress

In June 1995 the first Partial Birth Abortion Ban Act (HR 1833) was introduced in Congress to make it a federal crime to perform "an abortion in which the person performing the abortion partially vaginally delivers a living fetus before killing the fetus and completing the delivery." In March 1996 the House passed a revised Senate version that provided, in part:

(a) Whoever, in or affecting interstate or foreign commerce, knowingly performs a partial-birth abortion and thereby kills a human fetus shall be fined under this title or imprisoned not more than two years, or both.

(b) . . . the term partial-birth abortion means an abortion in which the person performing the abortion partially vaginally delivers a living fetus before killing the fetus and completing the delivery. . . . it is an affirmative defense . . . that the partial-birth abortion was performed by a physician who reasonably believed (1) the partial-birth abortion was necessary to save the life of the mother; and (2) no other procedure would suffice for that purpose.

In April 1996 President Bill Clinton vetoed the bill at a White House press conference at which five women described how they had made the decision to terminate their pregnancies with what could be considered partial birth abortions under the proposed law. He said that the debate was "not about the prochoice/prolife debate" but about the tragic circumstances of "a few hundred Americans every year who desperately want their children." Clinton made it clear that he would sign a bill that was consistent with *Roe v. Wade.* In the president's words, "I will accept language that says serious, adverse health consequences to the mother. Those three words."[5]

When the Senate voted in September 1996 to sustain the president's veto, the leader of the fight to override it was Senator Rick Santorum (R.-Pa.), who was challenged as having no personal experience or expertise in this area. A week after the unsuccessful vote, Senator Santorum had his own story to tell.[6] The senator's wife was pregnant with their fourth child when they were informed that ultrasonography showed their child had a "fatal defect," which turned out to be complete urinary tract obstruction. They were given three options: abortion, do nothing, or do in utero surgery to insert a shunt. They chose the shunt procedure, which was successfully performed at 20 weeks' gestation. The procedure resulted in an infection that put Karen Santorum in serious danger. An abortion would have removed the source of her infection, but she refused. Instead, she went into labor and gave birth to an extremely premature infant, Gabriel. Two hours later he died in his parents' arms.

This gave Senator Santorum the personal experience to make him a more credible antiabortion advocate. But his experience also illustrates at least two major problems with the partial birth abortion legislation he supports. First, his wife's actions can be considered praiseworthy only because she had a choice that is protected by current law. Second, the distinction between premature delivery and abortion at the edges of viability has always been problematic. Senator Santorum, for example, has been quoted as having said, in relation to this experience, that even when the life of the mother is at stake and "you have to end a pregnancy early . . . that does not necessarily mean having an abortion. You can induce labor, using a drug like Pitocin."[7] If one accepts the standard medical definition of abortion (termination of a pregnancy when the fetus is not viable), this distinction makes no practical sense: whether a planned abortion is performed or labor is induced, both are done to terminate a nonviable pregnancy. The real issue is not the method used to terminate the pregnancy, but the justification for terminating it. It is also reasonable to conclude that after the fetus is viable, abortion is simply no longer possible by definition; the only option is premature delivery.

What makes the term "partial birth abortion" so politically powerful is its inaccurate conflation of two polar opposite results of pregnancy, birth and abortion. Senator Daniel Patrick Moynihan (D.-N.Y.), for example, described it as "as close to infanticide as anything I have come upon."[8] But close is not identical. When Virginia attorney general Mark Earley describes the procedure as a "disturbing form of infanticide," he is making a legally inaccurate political statement. As the Supreme Court has repeatedly held, if a viable fetus is killed for the sake of the woman's life or health, the act is not infanticide by definition.

In January 1997 Senator Santorum reintroduced the Partial Birth Abortion Ban. At about the same time the executive board of the American College of Obstetrics and Gynecology (ACOG) issued its first and only statement on what it termed "intact dilatation [dilation] and extraction." The board wrote that it understood that the bill attempted to outlaw a procedure containing all of the following four elements:

1. deliberate dilatation [dilation] of the cervix, usually over a sequence of days;
2. instrumental conversion of the fetus to a footing breech;
3. breech extraction of the body excepting the head; and
4. partial evacuation of the intracranial contents of the living fetus to effect vaginal delivery of a dead but otherwise intact fetus.

The board described this as "one method of terminating a pregnancy" after 16 weeks. The board noted that it was sometimes used to save the life or

health of the mother, but that its "select panel . . . could identify no circumstances under which this procedure . . . would be the only option to
save the life or preserve the health of the woman . . . [although it] may be
the best or most appropriate procedure." The board's primary point was
that only the woman's physician should make the decision about what
particular procedure to use in individual circumstances, and that "the intervention of legislative bodies into medical decision making is inappropri-
ate, ill advised, and dangerous."[9]

The American Medical Association (AMA) took a different position.
On the eve of the Senate vote in May 1997, the AMA's board of trustees
agreed to support the legislation if Senator Santorum would add some
physician-friendly amendments.[10] State partial birth abortion bans are based
on the inherent police powers states have to protect the health and safety
of the public. The federal government has no such power, and the federal bill is based on the power of Congress to regulate interstate commerce. Because the AMA endorsed the federal bill, it implicitly agreed
that what physicians do with individual patients in their offices is a matter of interstate commerce. This is a stunning concession, because there
is no other area of medicine regulated by the federal government absent
federal funding.

Attempts to reach a compromise were made primarily by Senators
Dianne Feinstein (D.-Cal.), Barbara Boxer (D.-Cal.), and Thomas Daschle
(D.-S.D.). The Feinstein-Boxer amendment would have specifically dealt
with the *Roe v. Wade* problem the president had with the original bill by
adding "serious adverse health consequences to the woman" as an additional exception to the prohibition. Senator Daschle offered to ban all
abortions, by any technique, after viability except to save the life of the
pregnant woman or to protect her from "grievous injury" to her physical
health defined as "a severely debilitating disease or impairment specifically
caused by the pregnancy, or an inability to provide necessary treatment
for a life-threatening condition."[11]

Daschle's bill defined the realm of the debate as postviability (roughly
the third trimester) but nonetheless attempted to limit the reach of *Roe v.
Wade* by restricting the "health" of the pregnant woman exception to physical (not mental) health, and to risk of "grievous" harm at that. ACOG
endorsed the Daschle compromise, but in doing so it seemed to put politics over reasonable medical judgment, because the Daschle proposal limited the ability of physicians to act to protect their patients from harm, not
just from grievous harm.

In May 1997 the Senate adopted the Santorum bill 64 to 36, and in
October 1997 it was passed by the House and sent to the president. Two

days later President Clinton again vetoed the bill. He issued a three-paragraph message to the House of Representatives that said he was vetoing the bill "for exactly the same reasons I returned an earlier substantially identical version . . . last year [failure to include an exception for "serious harm" to a woman's health]."[12] Attempts to override the veto were again unsuccessful, and it was not until 2003 that Congress passed a substantially similar law.

Partial Birth Abortion in the Supreme Court

In the meantime, the Supreme Court heard a case on the constitutionality of partial birth abortion laws, specifically one that had been enacted in Nebraska. When the Court heard a challenge to Nebraska's law, partial birth abortion statutes had been enacted in 30 states. All the appeals courts except one, the Seventh Circuit Court of Appeals, had found these laws unconstitutional, and the Seventh Circuit opinion rested on an extremely narrow interpretation of the law under review.[13] The major controversies surrounding partial birth abortion have centered on the proper way to define the procedure and whether physicians ever need to employ the procedure to protect the health of a pregnant woman. These issues came to the U.S. Supreme Court in the case of *Stenberg v. Carhart*.[14]

The Nebraska law provided that

> No partial birth abortion shall be performed in this state, unless such procedure is necessary to save the life of the mother whose life is endangered by a physical disorder, physical illness, or physical injury, including a life-endangering physical condition caused by or arising from the pregnancy itself.

Like the federal acts twice vetoed by President Clinton, the Nebraska law defined partial birth abortion as "an abortion in which the person performing the abortion partially delivers vaginally a living unborn child before killing the child and completing the delivery." The law further defined the phrase "partially delivers vaginally a living unborn child before killing the unborn child" to mean

> Deliberately and intentionally delivering into the vagina a living unborn child, or a substantial portion thereof, for the purpose of performing a procedure that the person performing such procedure knows will kill the unborn child and does kill the unborn child.

Violation of the law is a felony that carries a prison term of up to 20 years, a fine of up to $25,000, and automatic revocation of the physician's medical license.

Leroy Carhart, a Nebraska physician who performs abortions, sued in federal court to have the law declared unconstitutional. U.S. District Court Judge Richard G. Kopf reviewed abortion procedures in detail, and even included a drawing of female pelvic anatomy as an attachment to his opinion, before holding that the statute was unconstitutional because it endangered women's lives and health, and was void for vagueness because physicians could not know what conduct was proscribed in the law.[15] The Court of Appeals for the Eighth Circuit affirmed.[16] By a five-to-four vote, the Supreme Court found the Nebraska law (and all other partial birth abortions laws) unconstitutional. The decision was written by Justice Stephen Breyer, one of only two justices (the other is Justice Ruth Bader Ginsburg) who had not previously expressed an opinion in a major abortion decision. Justice Breyer's opinion is best understood as a straightforward application of the principles articulated in the 1973 decision of *Roe v. Wade* and the 1992 decision of *Planned Parenthood v. Casey* to the Nebraska law.

The Nebraska ban applied throughout pregnancy and had no exception to preserve a woman's health. Under *Roe* and *Casey*, the state of Nebraska had to demonstrate that outlawing partial birth abortions would further a legitimate state interest and would not place an undue burden on women. Because it is a criminal statute, what exactly the statute prohibited had to be clearly defined. In order to determine exactly what was and was not prohibited, Justice Breyer, like the trial court judge, devoted almost all of his opinion to describing and comparing various abortion procedures and comparing them with the language of the Nebraska law.

Justice Breyer introduced his descriptions of abortion procedures by stating that they may seem "clinically cold or callous to some, perhaps horrifying to others," but that he saw no other way "to acquaint the reader with the technical distinctions among different abortion methods and related factual matters upon which the outcome of this case depends." Justice Breyer noted that 90 percent of abortions are performed before 12 weeks gestational age [which obstetricians calculate from the first day of the last menstrual period], and almost all the rest between 12 and 24 weeks. Almost all second trimester abortions use dilation and evacuation (D&E), with variations depending upon gestational age. Breyer quoted an AMA report saying that at 13 to 15 weeks, "D&E is similar to vacuum aspiration except that the cervix must be dilated more widely because surgical instruments are used to remove larger pieces of tissue." After 15 weeks, because of the increased size of the fetus and the rigidity of its bones, "dismemberment or other destructive procedures are more likely to be required . . . to remove fetal and placental tissue." And after 20 weeks, "some physicians use intrafetal potassium chloride or digoxin to induce fetal demise . . . to facilitate evacuation."

Breyer then made a series of observations and factual conclusions that determined the outcome of the case. He found, first, that the various D&E procedures have in common the dilation of the cervix, removal of at least some fetal tissue using surgical instruments, and (after the 15th week) the potential need for dismemberment of the fetus. When dismemberment does occur, it typically occurs "as the doctor pulls a portion of the fetus through the cervix into the birth canal." Breyer continued by noting that a variation of D&E, which the physicians who testified at the trial referred to as "intact D&E," or dilation and extraction (D&X), is used at 16 weeks at the earliest, when vacuum aspiration is ineffective and the fetal skull is too large to pass through the cervix. D&X proceeds in two ways: if the fetus presents head first, the physician collapses the skull and then extracts the intact fetus through the cervix; if it is a breech presentation, the physician pulls the fetal body through the cervix, then collapses the skull and extracts the fetus.

Based on medical texts and the position of ACOG, Justice Breyer concluded that "intact D&E and D&X are sufficiently similar for us [the Court] to use the terms interchangeably." There are no accurate statistics on the number of D&X abortions done in the United States, and Breyer cited estimates ranging from 640 to 5000 a year. Breyer found that D&X is performed for a variety of reasons, including reducing dangers from sharp bone fragments passing through the cervix, minimizing the number of surgical instruments used (and thus decreasing the likelihood of uterine perforation), reducing the likelihood of infection, and helping to assure the removal of all fetal tissue. D&X is also the preferred method for hydrocephaly and other anomalies incompatible with fetal survival.

This is much more detail of a medical procedure than has ever been seen in a Supreme Court opinion. The factual considerations, however, were necessary to answer the two major constitutional questions posed by Nebraska's statute: (1) Must a law prohibiting the use of a medical procedure for abortion contain an exception to protect the health of the pregnant woman as defined in *Roe*? And (2) does the Nebraska law "unduly burden" a woman's right to choose to terminate her pregnancy as defined in *Casey*? Justice Breyer's answer to both of these questions was yes.

Justice Breyer recited the rule in *Roe v. Wade* that a state may outlaw abortion after fetal viability to promote its interest in protecting potential human life, "except where it is necessary, in appropriate medical judgment, for the preservation of the life or health of the mother." Justice Breyer logically concluded that if *Roe* requires a health exception after viability, it certainly must require one before viability (when the state's interest in protecting fetal life is less).

Would the ban actually adversely affect the health of pregnant women who want to terminate their pregnancies? Justice Breyer concluded that it would, based on the record that demonstrates that "significant medical authority supports the proposition that in some cases, D&X would be the safest procedure." Breyer found especially persuasive the ACOG brief that stated that dilation and extraction "may be the best or most appropriate procedure in a particular circumstance to save the life or preserve the health of the woman." Nebraska relied on a contrary statement of the AMA that "there does not appear to be any identified situation in which intact D&X is the only appropriate procedure to induce abortion."

Breyer also rejected the argument that the word "necessary" in the phrase from *Casey*, "necessary, in appropriate medical judgment, for the preservation of the life or health of the mother" means an "absolute necessity" or requires "absolute proof." He concluded that the words "'appropriate medical judgment' must embody the judicial need to tolerate responsible differences of medical opinion." Breyer, who has special expertise in administrative law and risk assessment, continued, "the division of medical opinion about the matter at most means uncertainty, a factor that signals the presence of risk, not its absence." He concluded, "Where substantial medical authority supports the proposition that banning a particular abortion procedure could endanger women's health, *Casey* requires the statute to include a health exception when the procedure is 'necessary, in appropriate medical judgment, for the preservation of the life or health of the mother.'"

The second constitutional issue is whether the statute imposes an undue burden on a woman's liberty to terminate her pregnancy prior to fetal viability. The answer to this question depends on whether the statute is written precisely enough to apply only to the rare D&X procedures, and not to the much more routine D&E procedures as well. Based on medical descriptions of the various procedures, Breyer concluded that the language in the statute "does not track the medical differences between D&E and D&X."

Breyer thought it would have been a relatively simple matter for the state legislature to clearly articulate the differences between these procedures, but given the medical material he quotes in his opinion, it is very difficult to see how this could have been done. The attorney general of Nebraska, for example, argued unpersuasively that the two procedures were actually distinguished by the words "substantial portion" of the fetus, which the attorney general interpreted as meaning "the child up to the head" and thus not including "a fetal arm or leg or anything less than the entire fetal body." Because of the vagueness of the statute, Justice Breyer concluded that the statute was designed to put physicians using D&E in fear, because they "must fear prosecution, conviction, and imprisonment." Fear makes physcicians less likely to perform second trimester D&E procedures, and this places an undue burden on a woman's right to make a decision to have an abortion.

Justices John Paul Stevens, Sandra Day O'Connor, and Ruth Bader Ginsburg each wrote brief concurring opinions. Stevens emphasized that extreme antiabortion rhetoric tends to obscure the fact that over the past 27 years the core holding of *Roe v. Wade* "has been endorsed by all but 4 of the 17 Justices who have addressed the issue." He also argued (persuasively, I think) that "the notion that either of these two equally gruesome procedures [D&X and D&E after 15 weeks] performed at this late stage of gestation is more akin to infanticide than the other, or that the State furthers any legitimate interest by banning one but not the other is simply irrational." Justice O'Connor agreed with Breyer, but added that she thought "a ban on partial-birth abortion that only proscribed the D&X method of abortion and that included an exception to preserve the life and health of the mother would be constitutional." Justice Ginsburg emphasized that the Nebraska law would "not save any fetus from destruction" nor "protect the lives or health of pregnant women" and that therefore the state had no legitimate interest in enacting it. She also cited Chief Justice Richard Posner, who had made this point in a cogent dissent to the 7th Circuit opinion: "These statutes are not concerned with saving fetuses . . . [or] with protecting the health of women. . . . They are concerned with making a statement in an ongoing war for public opinion. . . The statement is that fetal life is more important than women's health."

The two major dissenting opinions were written by Justices Clarence Thomas and Anthony Kennedy (Chief Justice William Rehnquist joined both of them, and Justice Antonin Scalia joined the Thomas dissent). Justice Kennedy objected to the majority's use of medical texts and terminology to describe abortion procedures, arguing that this technical language "views the procedures from the perspective of the abortionist, rather than from the perspective of a society shocked when confronted with a new method of ending a human life . . . and may obscure matters for those not trained in medical terminology." He refused to refer to physicians as physicians, but rather called them "abortionists," and proceeded to describe the D&X procedure in lay terms, including: "with only the head of the fetus remaining in utero, the abortionist tears open the skull [using] . . . a pair of scissors." Kennedy concluded that permitting an exception to preserve the health of the woman would be the equivalent of forbidding Nebraska to ban partial birth abortions. In his words: "A ban which depends on 'the appropriate medical judgment' of Dr. Carhart is no ban at all."

Kennedy's central argument was that under *Casey*, states "have an interest in forbidding medical procedures which, in the State's reasonable determination, might cause the medical profession or society as a whole to become insensitive, even disdainful, to life, including life in the human fetus." But this argument could apply to all abortions and is not what *Casey* held. Moreover, he argued, it is irrelevant if the majority of the justices cannot see the difference between D&E and D&X abortions: "The issue is not whether members of the judiciary can see a difference between the two procedures. It is whether Nebraska can." Regardless of whether physicians can distinguish between medical procedures, Kennedy argued that the state of Nebraska has a "right to declare a moral difference" between two medical procedures.

Kennedy also believes there is a real difference, saying, among other things, "D&X perverts the natural birth process to a greater degree than D&E, commandeering the live birth process until the skull is pierced"; the fetus is "killed outside of the womb"; and D&X has a "stronger resemblance to infanticide." Finding that the state has a legitimate interest in outlawing this abortion procedure, Kennedy then argued that the Court has no medical expertise sufficient to second guess the legislature on its determination that D&X abortion is no safer than other abortion methods, and thus is never medically necessary. In this view, outlawing D&X abortions (which Kennedy believes is the only procedure that the statute can reasonably be read to outlaw) deprives no woman of access to a safe abortion, and thus cannot, under *Casey*, place an undue burden on the pregnant woman.

Justice Thomas, like Kennedy, was exasperated by Breyer's "sanitized" medical descriptions, noting that since *Roe*, "this Court has never before described the various methods of aborting a second or third-trimester fetus." Thomas also argued that the statute's plain language should be read only to include D&X abortions, and not D&E abortions. And to the argument that "partial birth abortion" is not a medical term, he replied simply (and accurately): "There is, of course, no requirement that a legislature use terminology accepted by the medical community." This left the issue of a woman's health. Thomas argued that the majority opinion "eviscerate[s] *Casey's* undue burden standard" because under the medical judgment test used by the majority, "there will always be some doctors who conclude that the [D&X] procedure is preferable." In his view, resolution of differences among physicians regarding the safety of abortion procedures should be left to the state legislatures. The dissenters, in short, simply do not believe that physicians can be trusted to make good faith decisions about the health of their patients.

Constitutional Law after Stenberg

The majority opinion in *Stenberg* took *Roe v. Wade* and *Casey* seriously. By applying the basic principles of these decisions, the majority found the Nebraska statute unconstitutional as an undue burden on a woman's right to choose an abortion under *Casey* because it was too vague (possibly covering D&Es and thus intimidating physicians into not performing them), and because it provided no exception for physicians to protect the health of the woman, as required by *Roe*. Five justices strongly reaffirmed *Roe* and *Casey* in *Stenberg*.

The somewhat surprising vote, and the one that has caused prochoice commentators the most concern, was that of Justice Kennedy, one of the three Justices (including Sandra Day O'Connor and David Souter) who wrote the joint opinion for the Court in *Casey*. Kennedy believed that the Nebraska law did not impose an undue burden on women under *Casey*, whereas O'Connor and Souter found that it did. Does this mean that Kennedy might change his mind about the *Casey* decision and vote to overrule it, along with *Roe v. Wade*, at some future time? No one can say for sure. But I did not believe this conclusion could be drawn from his dissent in *Stenberg* at the time, and any retreat from *Roe* and *Casey* by Kennedy seems even more unlikely after his sweeping majority opinion in *Lawrence v. Texas* applying the privacy principles of *Casey* to all adult sexual relations.[17]

The outcome in *Stenberg* was determined by *Roe* and *Casey*. Justice O'Connor may be correct that it would be possible to craft a statute that meets constitutional requirements. When Congress again passed a partial birth bill in 2003, a bill that President George W. Bush signed into law, the definition was rewritten:

(A) the person performing the abortion deliberately and intentionally vaginally delivers a living fetus until, in the case of a head-first presentation, the entire fetal head is outside the body of the mother, or, in the case of breech presentation, any part of the fetal trunk past the navel is outside the body of the mother for the purpose of performing an overt act that the person knows will kill the partially delivered living fetus; and

(B) performs the overt act, other than completion of delivery, that kills the partially delivered living fetus.[18]

Justice O'Connor might or might not find this definition sufficiently precise to overcome the vagueness problem. Even if she does (and she will probably be the deciding vote on this question), Justice Ginsburg remains correct that physicians would simply be required to pursue a different procedure to terminate the pregnancy. Thus, Senator (and physician) Bill Frist was simply wrong when he claimed after the Senate's 2003 64-to-34 vote that "the legislation we just passed will save lives." Many will, nonetheless, agree with him that the procedure described in the bill is one that "is barbaric, that is brutal, that is offensive to our moral sensibilities and it is out of the mainstream of the ethical practice of medicine today."[19] His statement also, of course, conflates health law and medical ethics.

The new law, like the one that Clinton vetoed, has no exception for the health of the pregnant woman. This seems to be consistent with the Bush administration's view of women—which is that it is much more important to protect fetuses than the health of pregnant women. This attitude was captured by photographers when President Bush signed the new partial birth abortion bill into law. In photographs of the signing that were displayed not just in the *New York Times*, but on the White House Web site as well, the president is surrounded by eight cheering middle-aged and elderly white male legislators. Apparently not one woman legislator could be cajoled into attending the signing of this unconstitutional and misogynistic law. Nor did the mini-crusade against women's rights end with the signing. When physicians sued to have the law declared unconstitutional, Attorney General John Ashcroft countered by attacking their women patients by demanding to see the medical records of every woman who had had an abortion performed by the physicians who questioned the law. As of mid-2004, the Attorney General's attempts to obtain private medical records have been unsuccessful, and the first court to hear a challenge to the law itself has (not surprisingly) declared it unconstitutional.[20]

President Clinton, who has consistently argued that abortion should be "legal, safe, and rare," was on strong constitutional grounds to base his vetoes on the failure of these bills to allow for physician action to preserve the pregnant woman's health. *Roe* requires an exception for the woman's health. Clinton was also on strong grounds in insisting, like ACOG, that the proper person to make a judgment about the health of the woman is the physician (of course, in partnership with the woman). As the Court put it in *Roe v. Wade*, this "decision vindicates the right of the physician to administer medical treatment according to his [*sic*] professional judgment."

Efforts to reframe the abortion debate always involve dichotomies that let us ignore or marginalize either women or fetuses by asking us to avert our attention from abortion itself and concentrate on something else. Most often this something else is the physician and the relationship of medicine to government. Other times it is (appropriately, I think) the pregnant woman and her life and health. Pregnancy is a unique human condition; there really is nothing like it in medicine or life, and we must therefore deal with it on its own terms, and not by analogy. This is simply impossible in the political arena but should not be impossible in the realm of personal decision making by pregnant women and their physicians.[21]

Medicine and Abortion

A deeper discussion of the necessity of safe abortion for women's lives and liberty may be too much to ask of either Congress or the Supreme Court. Maybe we are all past the point at which facts and logic matter in the abortion debate. As *Stenberg* underlines, the law can deal with whether abortions are permitted, but only physicians can determine how they can be safely and effectively performed. Ultimately, the most central question in abortion remains who makes the decision: the state, women, physicians, or women and their physicians together? The answer from the Supreme Court, as articulated in *Roe v. Wade* and its companion case, *Doe v. Bolton*, and strongly reinforced in *Stenberg*, is the woman and her physician together. In this respect the Court has been remarkably consistent in all the abortion cases—so much so that this conclusion is a principle of American constitutional law and American bioethics, near political hysteria notwithstanding. The much more meaningful and unsettled bioethics and health law issues in reproduction center on the new reproductive technologies, the topic I now turn to.

11

. . . .

The Shadowlands

Our impotence to craft an American ethics of abortion has led to a "Wild West" of unregulated research with human embryos and women by the reproductive medicine industry. Because of a "free for all" research mentality, it is becoming almost impossible to suggest outlandish and reckless possibilities for the new reproductive research without seeing them actually pursued by its practitioners. This is not only because there are no effective laws regulating the industry, but also because the bioethics of the field are exclusively focused on the potential parent–clients and have nothing to say about the potential children that are (or should be) the whole purpose for the field in the first place. As prepared as I am for the unexpected and bizarre in this field, even I was surprised when a respected American specialist, knowing that his research could not be ethically or legally performed in the United States, trained a Chinese student to pursue it in China. The results of this exercise in "ethical arbitrage" were announced in the United States with much fanfare at the annual meeting of the American Society of Reproductive Medicine and entered the annals of American bioethics.

The Chinese researchers took the nucleus from a dozen human oocytes (donated by a younger, fertile woman) and replaced them with the
nucleus of early embryos created using the "patient's" oocytes. This resulted
in "7 reconstituted zygotes, 5 of which developed to the 4 cell stage and
were transferred to the patient's uterus. The 5 embryos led to 3 pregnancies." The researcher continues the story:

> Fetal reduction to a twin pregnancy was performed transvaginally at
> 33 days post-transfer. At 24 weeks Fetus B delivered due to prema-
> ture rupture of membranes and died of respiratory distress. At 29
> weeks Fetus C delivered after intrauterine fetal demise due to cord
> prolapse. . . . Conclusion: Viable human pregnancies with normal
> karyotype can be achieved through nuclear transfer. . . . This finding
> suggests a unique approach to correct mitochondrial genetic disor-
> ders of maternal inheritance. Ongoing work to establish the efficacy
> and safety of nuclear transfer will result in its use as an aid for human
> reproduction.[1]

To label this a success and to state that it proves that this technique
will be established as an "aid for human reproduction" based on this seeming
slaughter of three "viable" fetuses seems ghoulish and totally ignores not
only the deaths of all three fetuses but the health and welfare of the pregnant woman as well. It is easy to see why this type of premature "trial and
error" research on fetuses is outlawed in the United States and it didn't
take China long to outlaw it as well.[2] What remains inexplicable is the inability of the reproductive medicine industry itself to set any limits at all to
the lengths American physicians can go, including going to other countries
to evade our very limited legal and ethical constraints, and putting women
and fetuses (as well as the health of the children who might survive these
experiments) at substantial risk.

This crude case is just one example in a long line of questionable experiments and sometimes incomprehensible legal decisions that illustrate
the need for both national and international regulation of the industry. In
this regard, experience in the United States, perhaps more than in any other
country, is the most eloquent argument for an international treaty of the
type proposed in Chapter 4. But more than an international treaty outlawing specific "species-endangering procedures" such as germ line genetic
engineering designed to produce "super children" is needed: carefully
crafted national standards of care and a federal regulatory scheme are also
called for. Although the industry continues to try to avoid regulation, court
cases from California, New York, Tennessee, and Massachusetts all sug-

gest that existing practices are inadequate to protect the interests of clinic patients and their children.[3]

Parentless in California

The California case involved Luanne and John Buzzanca, who used in vitro fertilization (IVF) with donor eggs and donor sperm to create embryos. The embryos were subsequently implanted into a genetically unrelated woman (the "surrogate" mother) for gestation and childbirth. The Buzzancas intended to rear the resulting child as their own. Before the child, Jaycee, was born, the couple separated, and John wanted nothing to do with the child.

At a trial to determine the legal parents of Jaycee, the identity of the genetic parents remained secret, and the gestational mother disclaimed any interest in the child. Because neither John nor Luanne was genetically or biologically related to Jaycee, the trial court judge concluded that Jaycee was parentless. As I characterized it at the time, this conclusion, that a child with six potential parents (assuming the surrogate mother was married) was legally parentless, was simply "stupid."[4] The decision was quite properly reversed on appeal.

The appeals court decided that because, under California law, a husband who consents to his wife's artificial insemination becomes the legal father of the child, "a husband and wife [should be] deemed the lawful parents of a child after a surrogate bears a biologically unrelated child on their behalf . . . [because] in each instance a child is procreated because a medical procedure was initiated and consented to by intended parents." Thus, the court concluded that Luanne and John were Jaycee's legal parents.[5]

To make sure no one missed the analogy, the appeals court later expanded on it, saying that gestational surrogacy and artificial insemination are "exactly analogous in this crucial respect: both contemplate the procreation of a child by the consent to a medical procedure of someone who intends to raise the child but who otherwise does not have any biological tie." The court didn't like the idea of people who are responsible for the creation of a child "turning around and disclaiming any responsibility after the child is born." Because the court believed that John "caused" the birth of Jaycee simply by signing a contract, the court had no problem concluding that the same logic that makes him the "father" makes Luanne (his wife at the time the surrogate mother contract was signed) the "mother," since she agreed to the "procreative project" at its inception.

The appeals court nonetheless concluded that it would be preferable for the legislature to set the rules in this arena: "we still believe it is the Legislature . . . which is the more desirable forum for lawmaking." And at the very end of the opinion the court tried to reassure John, now the legal father, that things might work out for the best. The court conceded that John may have agreed to the surrogate mother arrangement simply "as an accommodation to allow Luanne to surmount a formality," but observed that "human relationships are not static; things done merely to help one individual overcome a perceived legal obstacle sometimes become much more meaningful." Of course, there is no legal basis for such musings, and the court resorted to quoting literature to bolster its opinion. It referred approvingly to *Shadowlands*, a play about the life of C. S. Lewis and his marriage to an American citizen, Joy Gresham, which was arranged so that she could stay in England.[6] Just as a deeper relationship developed between Lewis and Gresham, the court seemed to be saying that a deeper relationship might develop between John and Jaycee, if not between John and his former wife, Luanne.

Frozen Embryos

On the other side of the country, the New York case involved an attempt by Maureen Kass and her husband, Steven, to become pregnant by IVF. In this attempt, Maureen had undergone five egg retrieval processes and nine embryo transfers, none resulting in a live birth. Prior to what turned out to be the tenth and final attempt, for which Maureen's sister agreed to try to carry the couple's embryos, the couple signed a series of four consent forms. Included in an addendum to one of the forms was a determination that if the couple "no longer wish to initiate a pregnancy or are unable to make a decision regarding the disposition of our stored, frozen prezygotes . . . [they] may be disposed of by the IVF program for approved research investigation as determined by the IVF program." After Maureen's sister failed to become pregnant, the couple decided to divorce.

Maureen then sought sole custody of the remaining frozen embryos so that she could undergo another implantation procedure. Steven opposed her request. The trial court granted custody of the embryos to Maureen, but an appeals court reversed in a split decision, a plurality deciding that the provision in the consent forms that provided that the embryos be turned over for research should be enforced.[7] The case was further appealed to New York's highest court, the Court of Appeals, which affirmed the decision that the couple's prior agreement should govern. The basic reason for its conclusion was: "advance directives, subject to mutual change of mind that must be jointly expressed, both minimize misunderstandings and maximize procreative liberty by reserving to the progenitors the authority to make what is in the first instance a quintessentially personal, private decision." If a document evidences informed, mutual consent, it should be honored by the courts. In the court's concluding words:

> As they embarked on the IVF program, appellant and respondent—"husband" and "wife," signing as such—clearly contemplated the fulfillment of a life dream of having a child during their marriage. The consents they signed provided for other contingencies, most especially that in the present circumstances the pre-zygotes would be donated to the IVF program for approved research purposes. These parties having clearly manifested their intention, the law will honor it.[8]

The court treated the consent form as a type of "Ulysses contract," an agreement that has as a major condition the prospective relinquishment of a right to change one's mind. Ulysses was warned by Circe to take precautions if he wanted to hear the Sirens' song, or there would be "no sailing home for him, no wife rising to meet him, no happy children beaming up at their father's face." So Ulysses ordered his men to bind him firmly to the mast, and instructed them that if he pleaded to be set free, they should bind him tighter still. But can a Ulysses contract have any real application to agreements about embryos?

The Massachusetts Supreme Judicial Court does not think so. The Massachusetts case involved a dispute in a divorce over the disposition of frozen embryos the couple had created in conjunction with IVF treatment. The wife wanted to use the embryos to attempt to have a child; the husband objected to this use. The couple was married in 1977, when they were both in the armed forces. They attempted IVF from 1988 through 1991, culminating in 1992 with the birth of twin girls. During this period two vials of embryos were frozen for possible future use. At the time of their divorce, one vial, containing four human embryos, remained in storage. The husband asked the probate court to permanently enjoin his wife from using the remaining embryos.

The probate court found that both husband and wife had signed a form entitled "Consent Form for Freezing (Cryopreservation) of Embryos" each time that cryopreservation was employed. The form listed various contingencies, such as death or separation, and asked the couple to determine what should be done with their remaining frozen embryos in these circumstances. The husband always signed a blank form, which the wife later filled in and also signed. She always specified that in the event of separation they "both agree[d] to have the embryo(s) . . . return[ed] to [the] wife for implant." The probate court concluded that the agreement was unenforceable because of "changes in circumstances" occurring in the four years since the form had been signed. These changes included the birth of twins, the wife obtaining a protective order against the husband, the husband filing for divorce, and the wife seeking to use the embryos to have additional children. In the words of the probate court, "no agreement should be enforced in equity when intervening events have changed the circumstances such that the agreement which was originally signed did not contemplate the actual situation now facing the parties." The wife appealed. The Massachusetts Supreme Judicial Court agreed that the contract should not be enforced.

The core of the opinion is the court's belief that courts should not enforce "agreements to enter into familial relationships (marriage or parenthood)," even if (unlike this contract) the contract is unambiguous and is signed with full knowledge by both parties. "As a matter of public policy, we conclude that forced procreation is not an area amendable to judicial enforcement," and courts "will not enforce contracts that violate public policy." The violation of public policy involves enforcing certain types of agreements that bind individuals "to enter or not to enter into familial relationships." For example, courts will not enforce agreements to marry, nor may any mother (in Massachusetts) agree to surrender her child until the fourth day after birth. Quoting from a prior opinion, in which the court refused to require a woman to continue her pregnancy at her husband's insistence, the court continued, "We would not order either a husband or a wife to do what is necessary to conceive a child or to prevent conception, any more than we would order either party to do what is necessary to make the other happy."[9]

The creation of human embryos for research purposes has always been contentious. Current U.S. law, for example, explicitly prohibits federal funding for the creation of human embryos for research purposes or any research in which human embryos are destroyed or discarded.[10] My colleagues Sherman Elias and Arthur Caplan and I have suggested that limiting embryo research to spare or surplus embryos from IVF clinics is a reasonable *political* compromise for obtaining federal funding.[11] The ethical basis for this political compromise is that these embryos were created for the legitimate purpose of procreation, and when this purpose is no longer sought by the gamete donors, destruction, donation, or research are the only alternatives. The choice of donating spare embryos for important medical research that cannot be done by other means is ethically superior to either destroying them or keeping them perpetually cryopreserved.

The National Institutes of Health (NIH) regulations drafted under the Clinton administration but put on hold by President George W. Bush would not only have required IVF clinics to have special rules for obtaining consent for use of surplus embryos for research, but also provided that:

- No inducements, monetary or otherwise, can be offered for the donation of embryos for research;
- There should be a clear separation between the decision to create embryos for infertility treatment and the decision to donate early human embryos in excess of clinical need for research purpose;
- Only frozen early human embryos should be used, and couples should be approached about donation only at the time of deciding the disposition of the excess embryos.[12]

The NIH guidelines thus would prohibit Ulysses-type contracts by implicitly requiring the contemporaneous consent of both gamete donors to use of surplus embryos for research (although the consent of the couple for research use sought at the time the embryos were no longer needed for reproduction could arguably remain in effect indefinitely) under the guidelines. They also go further in requiring that, like fetal tissue research, "to avoid possible conflicts of interest, the attending physician responsible for the fertility treatment and the researcher or investigator deriving and/or proposing to utilize human pluripotent stem cells should not [be] one and the same person."

Lessons

These cases from California, New York, and Massachusetts illustrate the two primary ways reproductive medicine clinics and courts have tried to avoid the new legal issues raised by new reproductive technologies: application of the sperm donor model of secrecy to all aspects of infertility treatment, and dependence on contracts. Both clinics and courts like contracts because enforcing contracts seems to put private, procreation-related decision making in the hands of the married couple and permits the court to simply interpret and enforce voluntary agreements. The problem, however, is that much more than contract law is at stake in these cases. Courts are not simply affirming the content of a contract, they are making much more profound and wide-ranging decisions about the status of embryos, the interests of children, and the identification and responsibility

of their parents. This is why, for example, no court has specifically enforced surrogate mother contracts, custody contracts, or marriage contracts by requiring that the parties to these contracts be bound by their
terms regardless of their current wishes or the best interests of the children involved.

The California court seems to be simply honoring an agreement made
before Jaycee's conception. But, in fact, the court is implicitly holding that
the determination of motherhood should be governed by the same rules
that the legislature has adopted to determine fatherhood in the case of sperm
donation. The court seems to see this as an example of gender neutrality,
but applying the male model of sperm donation to pregnancy and childbirth devalues both pregnancy and childbirth. This is because in the court's
analysis, not only the genetic mother (who as a donor of the ova used in
the "procreative project" could arguably be treated like a sperm donor,
even though donating ova is much more painful and risky than producing
sperm), but also the gestational mother is eliminated from consideration as
the child's mother. Likewise, the court simply accepts that because sperm
donors have historically had their identities kept secret even from the resulting children, therefore keeping the identity of both the ova donor and
the gestational mother a secret is reasonable.

Because both the primacy of contract and the value of secrecy can be
sensibly disputed, it is perhaps not surprising that the court concluded its
opinion with reference to *Shadowlands* rather than to the law. *Shadowlands*
is a strong play, and its main character, C. S. Lewis, was an insightful writer.
However, to cite the play for the proposition that "a deeper relationship"
may develop between a man and a woman than that contemplated at the
time of a marriage of convenience misses the point not only of the play
itself (which is about the meaning of suffering) but also of the case itself (in
which the marriage has already ended in divorce). For Lewis, the real world
is no more than "the shadowlands" from which we will emerge, like Plato's
cave-dwelling prisoners, into the afterlife.[13]

The California court's most significant insight is that courts have an
extremely difficult time making meaningful public policy in the realm of
assisted reproduction because they are limited to deciding individual disputes after the fact. The legislature, which ideally can foresee and prevent
disputes, is the preferred law-making body in this arena.

The New York court does not do much better. It seems to be especially proud of itself in affirming the contract–consent form the couple had
signed (even though it was a technical, boilerplate form that was difficult
to understand). But in affirming the contract, the court failed to examine
the public policy implications of its terms. For example, although informed

consent is necessary for human embryo research, the gamete donors retain the right to withdraw their consent at any time. To the extent that the
consent of both parties was necessary for valid consent to research (and
this is what the consent form required), the withdrawal of consent by either should mean that research cannot proceed. It may be that the court
missed this point because it adopted the language of the consent form, with
its meaningless term "pre-zygote" (instead of embryo). Other clinics have
used "pre-embryo," but virtually everyone has now abandoned the "pre"
designation because of the realization that the most meaningful distinction
is between extracorporeal embryos, over which both male and female gamete providers have equal say, and implanted embryos, over which the
pregnant woman has the ultimate decision-making authority. The terms
employed often determine the outcome, and it is evidence of the court's
confusion that even though the court says it is adopting the terms used in
the consent form, in the opinion itself the court uses three different terms
for the same entities: embryos, fertilized eggs, and pre-zygotes.

Finally, to the extent that the court is correct in concluding that the
couple embarked on IVF and signed the form "clearly contemplating the
fulfillment of a life dream of having a child during their marriage," their
divorce put an end to this dream and radically altered their circumstances.
Divorce, it would seem, should be a sufficient change to at least call the
embryo agreement, like the marriage agreement itself, into question, and
to provide each former spouse with the opportunity to revoke it. In this
regard the Massachusetts decision seems more reasonable.

These courts arguably did as well as they could, and reliance on
prior contract as a way to resolve controversies in assisted reproduction
has been espoused by some legal commentators as well. Nonetheless, the
California court seems correct in asking the legislature to establish rules for
the industry. The court's opinion, for example, gives no guidance as to
what would or should happen if the surrogate mother or the ovum donor
changed her mind and wanted to be designated the legal mother, with the
rights and responsibilities to rear Jaycee. Must obstetricians and hospitals
locate and interpret contracts to determine who a child's mother is at the
time of birth? Do commerce, money, and contracts really have more to
say about motherhood than do pregnancy and childbirth? If we take the
best interests of children more seriously than the best interests of commerce,
for example, children would be best protected by a universal rule that presumed that the woman who gave birth to the child was the child's legal
mother—with, among other things, the right to make treatment decisions
for the child and the responsibility to care for the child.[14] This is not because this is the traditional or natural rule; this is because the gestational

mother is the only one of the three potential mothers who we know will be present at the child's birth, and available to make decisions on behalf of the child. Treatment and care decisions must often be made immediately for the child; the issues of long term care, relinquishment of parental rights, and adoption can be dealt with later.

The New York Task Force on Life and the Law produced the first comprehensive legislative report on assisted reproduction in the United States,[15] which followed by more than a decade similar reports in the United Kingdom,[16] Australia,[17] and Ontario,[18] as well as a later report in Canada.[19] The United States has been slow to regulate the reproductive medicine industry because of continuing controversies over abortion and embryo research, and a basic belief that, to a large extent, couples and their physicians should be able to make their own decisions. Nonetheless, the tide against regulation may be turning. Procreative decisions are private, but certain aspects of them have such a profound impact on societal issues—such as the welfare of children, the social identity and responsibility of parents, basic informed consent requirements, and record keeping—that they require public scrutiny and regulation.

The reproductive medicine industry caters to the wishes of adults, and their wishes consistently trump the interests of the resulting children. The abortion model has been used to resist regulation (even though what is sought is a child, not the termination of a pregnancy), and the male sperm donor model has been consistently applied to ova donation, pregnancy, and childbirth, even though none of these are equivalents. Perhaps the most disturbing application of the male sperm donor model to virtually all assisted reproductive techniques is its allegiance to secrecy to such an extent that records about the sperm donor and the donation are routinely kept from the resulting children, who are systematically and consciously deprived of knowledge of their genetic parents. Secrecy has been the norm in donor insemination since its introduction. Worse, parents may be counseled to lie to their children about their genetic heritage, even though family secrets can be toxic to the entire family.[20]

Depending upon how one counts, the New York Task Force recommended approximately 60 changes in professional standards and guidelines, 30 changes in state regulation of gamete banks, and 11 new state laws. It is not necessary to agree with all of these recommendations to appreciate the vastness of the field and the multiple possible regulatory points. The task force was concerned, for example, about the growing number of multiple pregnancies induced by fertility drugs and the implantation of multiple embryos, both of which can result in multiple births with their problems of prematurity, or fetal reductions. Although the task force ultimately could not agree on how to regulate this area, a market approach would require infertility clinics to pay the cost of at least neonatal intensive care unit treatment of such multiple births. The task force was also concerned with the lack of uniformity of standards and record keeping and variations in consent procedures and forms, counseling, screening, success reporting, ova donation, and embryo research.

The most important decision the task force made was to adopt a child-centered analysis that takes the protection of the interests of children seriously. The task force does this, for example, by giving children legally identifiable and responsible parents and requiring clinics to keep records on their behalf. The most important specific recommendation was that "New York law should clearly provide that the woman who gives birth to a child is the child's legal mother, even if the child was not conceived with the woman's egg." This rule would have entirely avoided the California dispute, since the gestational mother and her husband would have been Jaycee's legal parents and would have had to give her up through standard adoption procedures. The task force's recommendations could also have solved the Kass dispute, since it recommends that use of frozen embryos should always require the agreement of both gamete providers, thus giving each veto power.

The task force's report is most important for its attempt to move the regulation of assisted reproduction out of the "shadowlands" of private clinics and the public realm of private disputes (the courts) and into the light of democratic lawmaking and regulation (the legislature). Both the regulation of medicine and family relations have historically been dealt with as state law questions. Thus, it has been seen as reasonable for the states to handle these issues themselves and for the law to develop on a state-by-state basis. Nonetheless, to the extent that the new reproductive technologies have become big business and are more accurately characterized as commercial than as medical or family-related activities, regulation of their interstate commercial aspects on a national level is vital.

Other countries that have developed uniform standards for the infertility industry have had to appoint a committee or commission to study the area and make legislative recommendations. It seems likely that if we want to seriously consider uniform commercial standards in this country, a similar panel will have to be appointed by the president, with the specific charge of developing uniform regulatory standards for the reproductive medicine industry. The President's Council on Bioethics took a baby step in this direction in 2004 when it made a series of relatively feeble recommendations regarding data collection, reporting requirements, patient protection measures, and professional oversight. The panel properly, however, emphasized that it is critical to "Treat the child born with the aid of assisted reproductive procedures as a patient."[21]

States will, of course, continue to have jurisdiction over determining motherhood, fatherhood, child custody, and related family law issues. But national commerce standards could be developed in this arena, as we have developed them for organ transplantation. In this regard, the agenda of a national advisory committee on new reproductive technologies should include consideration of uniform national rules in at least the following areas: the content of informed consent in terms of the risks to parents and children; standard ovum and sperm donor screening and record-keeping requirements; the ability of the resulting child to learn the identity of his or her genetic and gestational parents; rules for research on human embryos; time limits on the storage of human embryos; a prohibition on the use of gametes of the deceased to produce children; and the addition of human ova and embryos to the list of human tissues that cannot be purchased or sold in the United States.

The number of embryos transferred to produce a pregnancy may also have to be regulated. The adoption of voluntary guidelines by the industry has had only marginal success in decreasing the number of triplets and higher-order multiple births, which still account for 8% of all IVF births, and thus for almost one-fourth of all IVF children born. The percentage of twins continues to rise and twins currently comprise one in three IVF births.[22] This means that 100 IVF pregnancies will result in the births of about 150 children, 90 of whom (or about 60% of all IVF children) will be twins, triplets, or more, all of whom are at higher risk of prematurity and other medical problems. Because multiple births can be harmful to children, and because the goal of almost all couples who use IVF is to have one healthy child, a general single embryo transfer rule may ultimately be the only solution.

C. S. Lewis believed that a "bad way" to write for children is as a "special department of 'giving the public what it wants.'"[23] Similarly, a bad way to protect children who are born as a result of the new reproductive technologies is to simply provide adults, whether in the United States or China, with what they want. Children are the *only* reason for the reproductive medicine industry to exist, and the interests of children should be the primary concern of the industry.

Ulysses had an admirable spirit of adventure, but in ignoring his family obligations, he is not to be admired. Because of his deceitfulness, we encounter Ulysses in Dante's *Inferno*, in the eighth circle of hell (for sins of fraud). There is the obvious fraud of the Trojan horse, but Dante also has Ulysses explain his love of adventure and how his ego overwhelmed his duty to his family:

> Not fondness for my son, nor any claim
> Of reverence for my father, nor love I owed
> Penelope, to please her, could overcome
> My longing for experience of the world.[24]

Like Ulysses, the cover story for enforceable contracts in IVF clinics has been that they are necessary to support this "family-building" business. The truth is that Ulysses embryo contracts support the IVF clinics and make their business easier to run, but they undermine both fundamental legal principles and sound research ethics. That is why they are no longer tenable.

In the area of reproductive medicine, American bioethics and American health law can usefully be viewed as preschool fraternal twins, with much to learn from the rest of the world.

12

. . . .

Waste and Longing

W aste is not always what it seems.[1] In his cold war novel *Under-world*, for example, Don DeLillo explores the multifaceted qualities of waste. "Waste," he notes, "is the secret history, the underhistory, the way archaeologists dig out the history of early cultures, every sort of bone and broken tool, literally from under the ground." And waste can also be transformed to money:

> They are trading garbage in the commodity pits in Chicago. They are making synthetic feces in Dallas. You can sell your testicles to a firm in Russia that will give you four thousand dollars and then remove the items surgically and mash them up and extract the vital substances and market the resulting syrupy stuff as rejuvenating beauty cream, for a profit that is awesome.[2]

It is probably a rare (and desperate) person who would sell his testicles, but it also seems strange to try to sell a baby's umbilical cord blood (sometimes termed placental blood) to the newborn's mother by charging her for collecting and storing it. What makes this waste product of childbirth suddenly valuable to both parents and the public? The answer is that umbilical cord blood has gained new status as a natural resource that could supply hematopoietic (blood cell forming) stem cells for use in cases that would otherwise require a bone marrow transplant. With this new status have come new marketing strategies, as new for-profit and not-for-profit corporations seek the cooperation of hospitals and obstetricians, and the consent of pregnant women, for the collection, storage, and use of cord blood. Study of the ethical issues related to cord blood banking is ongoing.[3] Examination of the legal and social policy issues regarding the collection, storage, and use of cord blood, including the hidden dangers of commercializing this "waste" product, is also required.

In 1998 a study of 562 transplants of hematopoietic stem cells in cord blood units to unrelated recipients indicated that "placental blood is a useful source of allogeneic hematopoietic stem cells for bone marrow reconstitution."[4] Allogeneic transplants may be even better than autologous transplants in leukemia, because a graft-versus-leukemia effect lessens the probability of a relapse. A 2001 study concluded that umbilical cord blood from unrelated donors who are not HLA-matched can be therapeutic in treating adults for life-threatening blood disorders.[5] Many questions remain, but these studies confirm the usefulness of umbilical cord blood in unrelated recipients for a variety of conditions. They have also encouraged this growing industry to collect and store umbilical cord blood. A central policy issue is whether obstetricians should encourage patients to store umbilical cord blood for their own use in the for-profit sector, or to donate cord blood for the use of others in the not-for-profit sector.

Umbilical cord blood is usually described as useful for stem cell "transplantation." This phrasing implies that the organ transplantation model should be adopted for collection of umbilical cord blood. Seeing similarity seems natural because historically bone marrow transplantation (the major source of stem cells) has itself been treated as analogous to organ transplantation. One reason for this is that in Massachusetts, where the first human kidney transplant involving a living, minor donor was performed in 1957, the treating hospital, Peter Bent Brigham, went to court to obtain court approval (and legal immunity from battery and negligence) for performing surgery on the minor kidney donor.[6] Beginning in 1973, when Boston hospitals began to use minor donors as sources of bone marrow, they decided to go to court for permission to take bone marrow from minors as well, thus adopting the organ transplant model for donor consent.[7] This made some sense, because even though marrow is quickly replenished, the donors did have to undergo general anesthesia, together with its risks. On the other hand, the hospital lawyers could have (more appropriately, I believe) used the analogy of blood transfusions and avoided prospective court approval altogether.

Whatever one thinks of using the organ transplant model for the invasive procurement of bone marrow, it makes more sense to think of umbilical cord blood collection as more akin to blood donation than to organ donation. Unlike live bone marrow donation between siblings, for example, there is no conflict of interest between the welfare of the donor and the recipient, and the collection of cord blood itself (usually done before the placenta is delivered) involves no physical risk to the donor, either mother or newborn.

Which model is chosen matters because it will make some actions seem natural and even legally necessary, and others seem simply wrong. The practices that we have come to accept for blood collection and transfusion are not the same as those we accept for organ transplantation. For example, we take special precautions to protect live organ donors from harm and (although there are exceptions) generally require that they have a close family relationship to the recipient before permitting them to donate. Likewise, we prohibit the purchase and sale of human organs because we think this puts donors at risk of potentially coercive monetary inducements, and also because we highly value the "gift relationship" in organ transplantation as a rare and praiseworthy altruistic event in medicine.[8]

Thus, if we adopt the transplant model for umbilical cord blood, we will likely focus on risks to the live donor and forbid commerce and sales. On the other hand, use of the transfusion analogy will lead us to consider risks to the donor as minimal or nonexistent, to consider commerce as possible, even if not preferable, and to place our emphasis on assuring the safety of the blood itself prior to its use in a recipient.[9] When and if the collection of cord blood seems medically reasonable as a routine matter, we would likely promulgate required request rules for public blood banking if we apply the organ donation model. Likewise, we could require obstetricians to inform their patients of the option of personal banking if we adopt the blood donation model, similar to the way elective surgical patients are informed about the option of banking their own blood prior to surgery. It seems to me that the organ transplantation analogy is dysfunctional and misleading, and that adopting the blood transfusion analogy may help us more properly conceptualize the real issues in cord blood collection, storage, and use, even though this may lead us to permit some commerce in cord blood. The blood model would also put the Food and Drug Administration, which has jurisdiction over the safety of human blood, in charge of regulating cord blood safety.[10]

Ownership and Consent

The most important and contentious issues in the legal realm are the interrelated issues of ownership and consent, privacy, and commercialism. The identity of the source (and thus most likely the owner) of cord blood must be determined because this is the person who has the legal authority to consent to its collection and use. As a matter of biological and genetic identity, cord blood can be said to belong to the newborn child. That is why it is often used to screen the newborn for various conditions and infections. Umbilical cord blood is also a waste product, like urine, feces, and the placenta itself. But now that value has been discovered in this waste, and recycling it increases its value, any assumption that the owner of the waste has no interest in it evaporates. In the case of the newborn (and the newborn's valuable waste products), the mother has the right and responsibility to make decisions for the child, and also has the right to make decisions about the child's property and medical treatment, consistent with the child's best interests. The consent of both parents is not legally necessary.

Hospitals also have the right to dispose of human tissues (such as blood and placentas) in a manner consistent with good hospital practice. When umbilical cord blood was seen as a useless waste product of childbirth, disposing of it in the same manner as other human tissue was reasonable.[11] But once umbilical cord blood is identified as valuable, that value must be explained to the mother and her permission obtained to use the cord blood in the manner desired by the physician or hospital. This does not mean that the mother owns her child's umbilical cord blood; it seems most reasonable to consider the child as the legal owner. But it does mean that the mother has decision-making authority over the disposition of umbilical cord blood, at least so long as her choices are consistent with both reasonable medical practice and her child's welfare. This is why, although it seems most reasonable to consider the child the donor and owner of umbilical cord blood, it has nonetheless seemed appropriate to consider the mother the donor for the purposes of informed consent.[12]

Fetal tissue donation also provides a useful analogy here. The woman does not own her dead fetus, but she has more interest in its disposition than anyone else. Accordingly, only she can consent to have fetal tissue used for research or therapy, and in the absence of her consent, the fetus must be buried or cremated. It is generally suggested that her consent be sought before the abortion and be ratified after the abortion.[13] In a research protocol, the consent form and procedure must also be approved by an institutional review board (IRB). The blood donation model can help here as well, since use of the organ transplantation model in fetal tissue research has put far too much emphasis on the fetus itself as the tissue donor. The fetus, after all, is not the research subject. Moreover, since the fetus is dead, it cannot be harmed by the research. It is the recipient of fetal tissue who is the research subject, and emphasis should be placed on protecting the recipient–subject in fetal tissue research, just as it should be when umbilical cord blood is used in research. The research subject is the recipient of umbilical cord blood; there is no medical risk to the baby whose umbilical cord blood is used, nor to the mother who consents to its use.

Privacy and Commercialism

Although there are no physical risks in collecting umbilical cord blood, there are significant privacy risks. If umbilical cord blood is used for research or therapy, it must be screened for a variety of diseases, including HIV, and probably for at least some genetic disorders as well. In the 1998 study, for example, tests for hemoglobinopathies "and other genetic disease were performed . . . on the basis of family history and ethnic background."[14] If the blood is linked to the donor, screening creates medical information about the child and could disclose the otherwise "secret history" of the mother as well. This leaves two choices: either the mother's consent to perform the screening tests and create this medical information must be obtained (and steps taken to later inform her of the test results and keep them confidential from others), or the umbilical cord blood must be stripped of all individual identifiers so that the blood is not linkable to its source. Consent and privacy are generic issues with all so-called DNA databanks and DNA sample collections, not just umbilical cord blood banks.[15]

Privacy is of special concern in collecting, testing, and storing umbilical cord blood because the source of the blood is a newborn. There is general agreement that no genetic testing should be done on children for diseases that will not manifest themselves until adulthood and for which there is no preventive intervention or treatment that must be done prior to adulthood for efficacy.[16] It is possible that some additional useful information about the safety of the umbilical cord blood sample could be gained by following the child as he or she develops. Nonetheless, such surveillance seems both unlikely as a practical matter and potentially dangerous to the child's personal and informational privacy. It has been suggested that linkability in research projects involving umbilical cord blood be maintained but that "appropriate firewalls" be constructed to protect personal identity. The best privacy policy for public umbilical cord blood storage, however, is to unlink the sample from all identifiers so that the blood can be freely tested without simultaneously testing the child and its mother. This policy would also prevent recipients or their families from trying to contact the donor for another donation in case of a relapse. Physicians who want to protect their patients' privacy should advise their patients against donating umbilical cord blood to a blood bank that retains patient identifiers.

Commercialism may affect umbilical cord blood collection in two significant ways. First, the physician or hospital that collects the umbilical cord blood may want to use it for their own purposes, for example, to try develop a commercially viable product or for a research project. In either case, the physician has a fiduciary obligation to inform the mother of the research use, as well as the possible commercial applications of the research, and to obtain her consent to use the cord blood in this manner.[17]

Commercialism's second notable impact has come from the establishment of for-profit companies that market their services directly to pregnant women, offering to store umbilical cord blood for a price. Most of these companies have Web sites, and some of their advertising is readily accessible via the Internet. The direct marketing approach raises the obvious issues of truth in advertising and exploitation of patients at a particularly vulnerable time. The frequently used term "biological insurance," for example, is misleading, since the probability of the umbilical cord blood being of use to a family with no history of blood disease approaches zero (approximately 1 in 20,000 for the first 20 years of life), and one's own stem cells may also be less effective than a donor's.[18]

One underlying legal question is the nature of the relationship between the woman's attending physician (who must collect or supervise the collection of the blood) and the company: is the physician, for example, acting as an agent of the company (in which case the company is responsible for the physician's actions and negligence), or as an independent contractor (in which case the company is not responsible for the physician's acts)? The companies seem to want to treat the physician as an agent of the patient. At least one company, Viacord, has asked the patient to sign an "informed consent and release" form in which in lengthy legalese the patient agrees (on behalf of herself and her child and everyone else) never to sue Viacord for anything. In the research setting such a waiver of rights violates existing federal research regulations. Even in the therapeutic setting, in which umbilical cord blood is stored for possible future use by siblings, no physician should be a party to any medical procedure, including the collection of umbilical cord blood on behalf of his or her patient, that requires the patient to waive any of her rights to competent professional and accountable care. To do so is a violation of the physician's fiduciary duty to the patient.

Some umbilical cord blood storage forms provide that if the storage fees are not paid, the blood becomes the property of the storage company. This inappropriately treats cord blood like a pawned watch. It is defensible to destroy umbilical cord blood samples if fees are not paid, the way frozen embryos have sometimes been destroyed after the couples who agreed to their creation and storage abandoned them. Embryos should never be used for reproduction or research without the couple's informed consent. But it seems reasonable to permit the storage facility to use the umbilical cord blood for stem cell research if it has been abandoned, at least if privacy is protected by having all identifiers stripped from the sample. Permitting the storage company to sell the umbilical cord blood to others for therapeutic use, on the other hand, would put the storage facility in a conflict of interest position with both the donor (who benefits, if at all, only if the blood is retained in storage) and also the recipient (who would want records kept of the donor).

As market medicine matures and efficiency replaces ethics as the touchstone of medical practice, we will probably see more schemes to transform medical waste into profit. These are not necessarily bad (recycling can even be good), but unrestrained by law, such schemes undermine important values, including autonomy and privacy. In the case of umbilical cord blood, the promise of future use by a family without a history of a disease that blood stem cells could be used to treat seems unrealistically excessive and deeply exploitive of vulnerable new parents. Americans, at least in the short term, will nonetheless most likely consider umbilical cord blood storage just another market choice that people can make or reject as they see fit, at least as long as they can pay for it. This is also how many physicians will likely see it as well: another waste product transformed into gold. Of course, the source of this gold could quickly change if a method is developed to expand pluripotent stem cells in vitro, so that virtually limitless supplies of stem cells could be created from a few progenitor cells. Until that time, however, the legal and policy issues in umbilical cord blood banking must be faced.

The transplant analogy, although somewhat misleading, could lead us to encourage altruistic donations to not-for-profit umbilical cord blood banks and to encourage communitarian values in this domain of medicine. There is a serious shortage of matched bone marrow for transplant, and public umbilical cord blood banks could help relieve it. This is the most responsible way to develop this new field. An entity similar to the United Network for

Organ Sharing (UNOS) should be authorized and funded by Congress so that American patients can benefit from this new source of stem cells.[19] The fact that anyone purchases this type of "biological insurance" also illustrates the fact that there is no limit to the amount of money some people will pay for any chance to increase the odds that they or their children might live longer. Americans fear death, and as a market good that promises a longer life, medicine has no price limit.

DeLillo would be pleased to learn of this new choice and of the longing for security and good health that it represents. But he would also likely remind us (and the new parents, the new companies, and the umbilical cord blood researchers) that "Most of our longings go unfulfilled. This is the word's wistful implication—a desire for something lost or fled or otherwise out of reach." But desires persist, nonetheless, and we now deal in birth and death simultaneously by creating children to provide cord blood stem cells to a dying sibling.

Savior Siblings

The first, and still the best known, case of a "savior sibling" is the story of Jack and Lisa Nash, and what the Colorado couple did in an effort to save their 6-year-old daughter, Molly, helps us better understand the continuing debate about human embryo and stem cell research.[20] Molly suffers from Fanconi's anemia and was expected to die of leukemia. The best hope for saving her life was an infusion of healthy, compatible stem cells. So the Nashes set out to provide a donor.

The couple, using in vitro fertilization and with the help of Chicago physicians, formed 15 embryos and, through preimplantation genetic diagnosis (PGD), identified those free of Fanconi's anemia. Then—in what was a medical innovation—they screened those healthy embryos again to see if any would produce stem cells that would be an HLA match for Molly. One match was found, and that embryo was implanted in Lisa Nash's uterus. Adam was born. Doctors in Minnesota took stem cells from baby Adam's umbilical cord blood and transplanted them into his ailing big sister in an attempt (so far successful) to replace the diseased stem cells in her bone marrow with healthy ones.

The Nashes engaged only in screening embryos that they produced, and all were at risk for Fanconi's anemia. There was no attempt to alter the genetic composition of the embryos. Their actions did not cross a new ethical line, although embryo screening itself raises important issues. Should

IVF and PGD be used for the sole purpose of obtaining an HLA-matched embryo when the embryos are not at risk for a genetic disease? Or would this use of medical technology, as Britain's regulatory agency has ruled, put the potential child at unwarranted risk?[21] Some American medical ethicists are already arguing that the risks are minimal, and we should not take slippery slope arguments seriously—at least not as long as the rationale for embryo screening is to try to save the life of an existing child. One physician-ethicist, Norman Fost, has even suggested that screening an embryo to produce a child to be a kidney donor should be praised.[22] This view puts us at the bottom of the slope to begin with by too easily accepting two propositions that are problematic: that it is acceptable to treat a child primarily as a means rather than as an end in itself; and that it is never legitimate for physicians to question the motives of potential parents. These propositions are radical, and help explain the continuing opposition to more reasonable uses of PGD.[23]

We have entered the realm of embryo research almost exclusively to treat existing diseases and disabilities; in vitro fertilization itself was developed to help couples who could not otherwise have children. And PGD has been used almost exclusively to identify embryos that would produce severely disabled children, and now—with the Nash case—also to help in the treatment of an existing terminally ill child. Likewise, destroying "left over" IVF embryos so that stem cells can be harvested from them and creating custom-made embryos by cloning have both been suggested only for therapeutic purposes: to grow tissue to use in treatment of diseases such as Parkinson disease and diabetes, and to tailor make such tissue so that it will not be rejected.

The general societal acceptance of embryonic stem cell research, and of the Nash family story, indicates that society supports embryo screening and embryonic stem cell harvesting for the purpose of curing or finding cures for serious diseases. This seems reasonable, given that embryos are not people (they are not even fetuses), cannot suffer, no pregnancy is involved when they are created in the laboratory, and their use in scientific research could lead to new ways to alleviate intense human suffering.

But it is a difference in kind rather than degree to try to re-engineer humans, and there is an understandable general revulsion to using our new-found genetic techniques to make "designer" babies or to try to improve upon the species by creating super babies. As discussed in Chapters 3 and 4, the first commodifies children and threatens to remake the parent–child relationship into a manufacturer–product relationship, and the second threatens to create a new type of human, a super- or subspecies, which could either destroy "standard-issue" humans or be destroyed by them if they are seen as a threat. The central question of those chapters is confronted again here: can our downhill incremental slide from preimplantation genetic screening of embryos to trying to genetically alter them be prevented? It will not be easy. Prevention will require prohibiting the genetic alteration of any human embryo destined to be used to start a pregnancy. We could, however, permit the production of cloned and genetically altered embryos for societally critical research and treatment—but only with effective public oversight.

Some object to this possibility because they think that the research and treatment exceptions would represent a step down a slippery slope and inevitably would lead to using these embryos to try to make babies. But that view ignores a social reality: the public will almost certainly demand that this research be done if it holds great promise to alleviate serious diseases—and it will be right to do so. Better to accept this reality and prevent sliding down the slippery slope by adopting and consistently enforcing a strict rule against starting a pregnancy with a genetically altered embryo.[24] Another objection to this possibility is that it would prohibit attempts to treat embryos affected with serious diseases. But treatment is likely to be dangerous for the resulting child, and in any event is inefficient; better to simply destroy the embryos with serious diseases, as was done in the Nash case, rather than perform such a radical experiment.

Moreover—and the slippery slope is much more of a danger here—if we permitted the genetic alteration of embryos for treatment, the skills developed in this activity would quickly be put to use for embryo enhancement because the line between treatment and enhancement is inherently ambiguous. One person's cure or prevention is another person's enhancement. A federal law (and, ultimately, an international treaty along the lines suggested in Chapter 4) prohibiting the use of any and all genetically altered human embryos to produce a pregnancy could erect a barrier on the slope toward genetically engineered children. Such a law (and treaty) would be a concrete manifestation of bioethics and human rights symbiosis.

Concluding Remarks

*Bioethics, Health Law, and Human Rights
Boundary Crossings*

In his compelling novel *Blindness*, José Saramago tells us about victims stricken by a contagious form of blindness who were quarantined and came to see themselves as pigs, dogs, and "lame crabs." Of course, they were all human beings—although unable to perceive themselves, or others, as members of the human community. The disciplines of bioethics, health law, and human rights are likewise all members of the broad human rights community, although at times none of them may be able to see the homologies, even when responding to a specific health challenge.

The boundaries between bioethics, health law, and human rights are permeable, and border crossings, including crossings by blind practitioners, are common. Two working hypotheses form the intellectual framework of this book: we can more effectively address the major health issues of our day if we harmonize all three disciplines; and American bioethics can be reborn as a global force by accepting its Nuremberg roots and actively engaging in a health and human rights agenda. That these disciplines have often viewed each other with suspicion or simple ignorance tells us only about the past. They are most constructively viewed as integral symbiotic parts of an organic whole.

A review of the bioethics topics addressed in this book and how they have been addressed in recent years underscores the close relationship between bioethics and human rights, especially as they are used in the new field of health and human rights, but more generally in the nongovernmental organization community, the developing world, and the academic community. Is the interest in globalization, public health, and human rights completely novel for American bioethics, or is it in fact a natural development in a field whose origins have been mostly misunderstood or suppressed? My tentative conclusion is that the evidence supports the latter view.

Both American bioethics and international human rights were born from World War II, the Holocaust, and the Nuremberg tribunals held in American-occupied Germany. While the Doctors' Trial was only a part of Nuremberg and the new field of international human rights law, I believe it is accurate to conclude that the trial itself marked the birth of American bioethics. At the Doctors' Trial, American judges articulated the Nuremberg Code of human experimentation based on the arguments of American prosecutors, and American physicians served as both consultant to the prosecution and expert witness in helping the court to articulate the code.[1]

Reaching this conclusion after exploring the variety of topics in this book suggests T. S. Eliot's fabled lines from *Little Gidding*:

> We shall not cease from exploration
> And the end of all our exploring
> Will be to arrive where we started
> And know the place for the first time.

It is coincidental, but fitting nonetheless, that T. S. Eliot composed these lines during World War II when he was a night fire-watcher during the fire bombings of London. World War II was the crucible in which both human rights and bioethics were forged, and they have been related by blood ever since. Recognizing and nourishing this birth relationship will permit American bioethics to break free from its focus on, if not obsession with, the doctor–patient relationship and medical technology and to cross our own border to become a global force for health and human rights—not as an imperialistic project, but to learn from and work with other cultures, countries, and activists.

In reflecting on the principled foundation of his philosophy, Descartes adopted a model from nature: "Philosophy as a whole is like a tree whose roots are metaphysics, whose trunk is physics, and whose branches, which issue from this trunk, are all the other sciences." Of the sciences themselves,

Descartes identified three principal ones, "medicine, mechanics, and morals." The fruits of this tree, Descartes went on to note, will only be culled from "the extremities of the branches" and what they will turn out to be may not be known until they actually appear.[2]

The tree metaphor works here as well. The human rights tree took root and was nourished in the blood and ashes of World War II and the Holocaust. Its roots are in universal law and human dignity, both of which apply to all humans by virtue of their humanity, and which were articulated at the trial of the major Nazi war criminals at Nuremberg. The trunk of this human rights tree is made up of the Nuremberg Principles, the Charter of the United Nations, and the Universal Declaration of Human Rights.[3] The branches are the major human activities needed to bring the human rights outlined in the Declaration to fruition. One of these branches is bioethics, and other branches include health law, international law, treaties, humanitarian law, corporate law, and corporate ethics. Science, technology, and economic development can also be seen as branches. The fruits of each branch will, of course, vary, some nourishing the mind, some the soul, and some the body.

Although the World War II origin of American bioethics seems obvious at the beginning of the 21st century, mainstream bioethics historians may continue to prefer seeing American bioethics as a 1960s–70s response to medical paternalism made more powerful by medical technology, especially organ transplantation and mechanical ventilation.[4] Moreover, there was an active program to bury the Nazi past and distance American medicine and American bioethics from Nazi medicine for fear it would be somehow tarnished by it.[5] The best-known example is probably Henry Beecher—sometimes credited with getting American bioethics started with his 1966 essay in the *New England Journal of Medicine* that catalogued unethical experiments.[6] Beecher was also a leader in drafting the Helsinki Declaration on human research—which he saw as a way to "save" medical research from becoming dominated by the Nuremberg Code.[7] Nuremberg was also on the minds of Daniel Callahan and the founders of the Hastings Center, and they held a major program on its implications for bioethics. But, as described by Arthur Caplan (who himself sponsored a similar program a decade later, in 1989), there were many reasons for American bioethics to suppress its birth, most notably the sheer unprecedented scale of immorality of the Nazi doctors and potential guilt by association, especially in the research enterprise.[8] Although he does not use the phrase in his book on the subject, I recall Caplan saying at this meeting, "bioethics was born from the ashes of the Holocaust."

The source of American bioethics can be read in the biographies of almost all of the founders of American bioethics and its current leaders.[9] But the history of American bioethics is rooted in the Nazi concentration camp in another way as well. Historians are correct to see American bioethics in the late 1960s and early 1970s as fundamentally a reaction to powerful new medical technologies in the hands of medical paternalists who disregarded the wishes of their patients. Thus, the major strategy to combat this unaccountable power was to empower patients with the doctrine of informed consent (sometimes called autonomy, and put under the broader rubric of respect for persons). This is perfectly reasonable. But it is unreasonable to want to distance yourself so much from your origins to miss the fact that Nazi physicians who performed experiments in the concentration camps did so in an impersonal, industrial manner on people they saw as subhuman, and were unaccountable in the exercise of their power over their subjects. The first response of the American judges to the horror of the Nazi doctors was to articulate, in the first precept of the Nuremberg Code, the doctrine of informed consent. The modern doctrine of informed consent was not born either of U.S. health law in 1972, or of American bioethics shortly thereafter, but at Nuremberg in 1947. Misidentifying the birth of bioethics has also helped us to misidentify the birth of its primary doctrine, informed consent. American bioethicists have spent so much energy denying their origins that they have produced a misleading account of their central doctrine as well. The American judges at Nuremberg were comfortable crossing borders, especially the border between American medical ethics (what we now know as bioethics) and international law.

As in any organic whole, the boundaries between these related fields are easily crossed, as the essays in this book suggest. The collapsing of other boundaries in human rights discourse suggests how a more integrative model might be built. In the brief history of human rights, for example, there have been three great divisions—all of which have been effectively breached (although attempts to police these borders persist). These are the divisions between positive and negative rights, between public and private actors, and between state internal affairs and matters of universal concern.[10]

The positive/negative distinction has been seen more and more as a difference in degree rather than kind. This is because positive government action is required even to ensure so-called negative rights such as the right to be left alone, the right to vote, freedom of speech, and the right to trial by jury. All of these negative rights actually require the government to do something positive—such as setting up a police and court system, and making legal counsel available to the accused. Of course, in the arena of positive rights, like the right to food, shelter, jobs, and health care, governments will be required to expend more resources to fulfill these rights. But resources will have to be expended to fulfill both types. In the language of contemporary human rights, governments don't simply have the obligation to act or not to act; but rather have obligations regarding all rights to *respect* rights themselves, to *protect* citizens in the exercise of rights, and to *promote* and *fulfill* rights. Of course, not all governments can fulfill economic rights immediately because of financial constraints, and international law suggests that governments must work toward the "progressive realization" of these rights within the limits of their resources, as discussed in the chapter on the right to health (Chapter 5).

A similar analysis can be made of the distinction between private and public. Individuals cannot be free to commit crimes in the privacy of their homes; the law has jurisdiction in both the public and private sphere. And although international law has traditionally focused solely on the relationships between governments (and between a government and its people), private actors, like transnational corporations, have more recently been seen as having so many direct relationships with governments, who often act explicitly to protect their interests, that they should be seen as a fit subject for international human rights. Similarly, although historically the boundary of a country protected it from interference with its "internal affairs," the world today will not always now simply stand by and watch as countries engage in massive human rights abuses (as the world did in Rwanda), but may rather, as in Bosnia, intervene to prevent major human rights abuses.

As mentioned a number of times in this book, in human rights work entirely new entities, termed nongovernmental organizations or simply NGOs, have sprung up and become the leading forces for change in the world. A notable health-related example is Médecins sans Frontières, (MSF) a humanitarian-human rights organization founded on the belief that human rights transcend national borders and thus human rights workers cannot be constrained by borders, but should cross them when necessary. As Renée Fox describes it, over the years the *le droit d'ingerence* (the right to interfere) has been displaced with an even more activist *le devoir d'ingerence* (the duty to interfere).[11] This concept, of course, takes human rights to be universal and sees globalization as a potential force for good. This physician organization thus redefines medical ethics as physician action to protect human rights, blending these two fields and treating law as subordinate to the claims of human rights. In this regard, MSF itself can be seen as one of the first health and human rights fruits of our human rights tree. Other notable physician NGOs include Physicians for Human

Rights, International Physicians for the Prevention of Nuclear War, and Global Lawyers and Physicians.[12]

Globally, boundaries are being breached even as the world paradoxically splinters into more and more countries. Nonetheless, as daunting and discouraging as many of the contemporary challenges discussed in this book can be, especially those related to global terrorism, the coming of the post-human, and provision of basic health care to everyone, the Universal Declaration of Human Rights really does provide the world with an agenda and a philosophy. The centrality of the UDHR to bioethics is well-recognized internationally. Stated concisely in a 2003 report of the International Bioethics Committee of UNESCO, "modern bioethics is indisputably founded on the pedestal of the values enshrined in the Universal Declaration of Human Rights."[13] The world's one remaining superpower and empire builder, the United States, has yet to embrace the Declaration—even though it was drafted under the able direction of Eleanor Roosevelt[14]—and has even turned itself into an object of fear and distrust around the world in the wake of our "preemptive war" in Iraq. This war, allegedly fought because of the threat of terrorism, also added a new dimension to bioethics discourse.

Before the war on terror, the paradigm that most American bioethicists, especially those on President Bush's Council on Bioethics, worried about was Huxley's *Brave New World*—a world in which humans would be commodified and stratified, and would give up all of their dignity and self-respect for security and recreational drugs and sex. It was a world of humans reduced to animal status.[15] These concerns have not disappeared with the twin towers, but they are now supplemented with a parallel concern, the warning outlined in Orwell's *1984*: a world dominated by dictatorships kept in power by fear induced by "perpetual war," debasement of language (doublespeak), and the constant rewriting of history.

Bioethics alone, of course, can effectively confront neither vision: one is dominated by private, corporate interests and nourished by desire and money, in essence, market-driven capitalism, making economics supreme. The other is fueled by the concentration of government power in a few people who want to maintain their power, meaning politics and law must be the foremost players. And, of course, all of this takes place in a newly globalized world in which time and space are compressed and information travels instantly. This is most easily visualized by the SARS epidemic, in which the virus traveled globally, crossing boundaries in days—but in which information about the virus traveled (and mutated) instantly and literally knew no national boundaries. While bioethics has aspired to be a universal language, the only language that can be said to have attained that status, as tentative as it is, is the language of human rights.[16]

A *Brave New World* soma and artificially "reproduced" future, one that could be brought into being by developments like genetic engineering (Chapters 3 and 4), new reproductive technologies (Chapter 11), and an appetite for immortality (Chapter 12), would strike at the roots of the human rights tree by shrinking our humanity and with it our "natural" rights. A *1984* dictatorship supported by perpetual war that sustains fear, one suggested by a new war on terror (Chapter 1) and continued obsession with state-sanctioned killing (Chapter 6), threatens to simply chop down the human rights tree, or at least to chop off major branches of it. The remaining chapters are primarily about fruits—including decent health care for everyone (Chapter 5), patient rights (Chapter 8), and reproductive choices (Chapter 10). The ultimate shape and taste of these fruits is unknown, as is the ultimate shape of the tree—including that part made up of the interrelationship of human rights with bioethics and health law. What is evident is that human rights activists are more likely to provide nourishment to the human rights tree than bioethics theorists or health law scholars.

Salman Rushdie also had border crossings on his mind when he reflected on the meaning of 9/11 in his collection entitled *Step Across This Line*. He ends his reflections by noting that "We are living, I believe, in a frontier time, one of the great hinge periods in human history, in which great changes are coming about at great speed." On the plus side, he lists the end of the cold war, the Internet, and the completion of the human genome; on the minus, a "new kind of war against new kinds of enemies fighting with terrible new weapons." The changes we will adopt are not preordained, and Rushdie quite properly notes that "the frontier both shapes our character and tests our mettle."[17] He is also right to wonder whether as we stand on this frontier if we will regress into barbarism ourselves or "as custodians of freedom and the occupants of the privileged lands of plenty, go on trying to increase freedom and decrease injustice?" A globalized American bioethics, infused with human rights, would have to pursue global justice.

In another post 9/11 reflection, José Saramago astutely agrees that what our world needs most of all is justice, "a justice that is a companion in our daily doings, a justice for which 'just' is most exactly and strictly synonymous with 'ethical,' a justice as indispensable to happiness of the spirit as food for the body is indispensable to life." Saramago has in mind not only a justice "practiced in the courts whenever so required by law" but more, "a justice that manifests itself as an inescapable moral imperative . . ."

Where do we find the embodiment of this universal justice that is required by law and nourished by ethics and moral imperatives? In Saramago's words "we already have a readily understandable code of practical application for this justice, a code embodied for the past fifty years in the Universal Declaration of Human Rights, those thirty essential, basic rights . . . in terms of the integrity of its principles and the clarity of its objectives, the Universal Declaration of Human Rights, just as it is now worded and without changing a single comma, could replace to advantage the platforms of every political party on Earth . . ."[18]

This is powerful language and clear eyed: Saramago is no romantic seeking a new Eden, but a realist who understands that without a human rights–focused action by both individuals and governments, "the mouse of human rights will implacably be eaten by the cat of economic globalization." Saramago's implicit assertion is that law, ethics, and human rights are all of a piece—and that justice cannot be obtained for humans without all three components.

American bioethics was born with international human rights law— and these branches of the human rights tree are much more likely to yield fruit, especially in areas like the right to health and rights in health, if their practitioners work together organically to fulfill the promise of its trunk, the Universal Declaration of Human Rights.

Appendix A

Universal Declaration of Human Rights

Preamble

Whereas recognition of the inherent dignity and of the equal and inalienable rights of all members of the human family is the foundation of freedom, justice and peace in the world,

Whereas disregard and contempt for human rights have resulted in barbarous acts which have outraged the conscience of mankind, and the advent of a world in which human beings shall enjoy freedom of speech and belief and freedom from fear and want has been proclaimed as the highest aspiration of the common people,

Whereas it is essential, if man is not to be compelled to have recourse, as a last resort, to rebellion against tyranny and oppression, that human rights should be protected by the rule of law,

Whereas it is essential to promote the development of friendly relations between nations,

Whereas the peoples of the United Nations have in the Charter reaffirmed their faith in fundamental human rights, in the dignity and worth of the human person and in the equal rights of men and women and have determined to promote social progress and better standards of life in larger freedom,

Whereas Member States have pledged themselves to achieve, in co-operation with the United Nations, the promotion of universal respect for and observance of human rights and fundamental freedoms,

Whereas a common understanding of these rights and freedoms is of the greatest importance for the full realization of this pledge,

Now, therefore,

The General Assembly,

Proclaims this Universal Declaration of Human Rights as a common standard of achievement for all peoples and all nations, to the end that every individual and every organ of society, keeping this Declaration constantly in mind, shall strive by teaching and education to promote respect for these rights and freedoms and by progressive measures, national and international, to secure their universal and effective recognition and observance, both among the peoples of Member States themselves and among the peoples of territories under their jurisdiction.

Article 1

All human beings are born free and equal in dignity and rights. They are endowed with reason and conscience and should act towards one another in a spirit of brotherhood.

Article 2

Everyone is entitled to all the rights and freedoms set forth in this Declaration, without distinction of any kind, such as race, colour, sex, language, religion, political or other opinion, national or social origin, property, birth or other status.

Furthermore, no distinction shall be made on the basis of the political, jurisdictional or international status of the country or territory to which a person belongs, whether it be independent, trust, non-self-governing or under any other limitation of sovereignty.

Article 3

Everyone has the right to life, liberty and security of person.

Article 4

No one shall be held in slavery or servitude; slavery and the slave trade shall be prohibited in all their forms.

Article 5

No one shall be subjected to torture or to cruel, inhuman or degrading treatment or punishment.

Article 6

Everyone has the right to recognition everywhere as a person before the law.

Article 7

All are equal before the law and are entitled without any discrimination to equal protection of the law. All are entitled to equal protection against any discrimination in violation of this Declaration and against any incitement to such discrimination.

Article 8

Everyone has the right to an effective remedy by the competent national tribunals for acts violating the fundamental rights granted him by the constitution or by law.

Article 9

No one shall be subjected to arbitrary arrest, detention or exile.

Article 10

Everyone is entitled in full equality to a fair and public hearing by an independent and impartial tribunal, in the determination of his rights and obligations and of any criminal charge against him.

Article 11

1. Everyone charged with a penal offence has the right to be presumed innocent until proved guilty according to law in a public trial at which he has had all the guarantees necessary for his defence.
2. No one shall be held guilty of any penal offence on account of any act or omission which did not constitute a penal offence,

under national or international law, at the time when it was committed. Nor shall a heavier penalty be imposed than the one that was applicable at the time the penal offence was committed.

Article 12

No one shall be subjected to arbitrary interference with his privacy, family, home or correspondence, nor to attacks upon his honour and reputation. Everyone has the right to the protection of the law against such interference or attacks.

Article 13

1. Everyone has the right to freedom of movement and residence within the borders of each State.
2. Everyone has the right to leave any country, including his own, and to return to his country.

Article 14

1. Everyone has the right to seek and to enjoy in other countries asylum from persecution.
2. This right may not be invoked in the case of prosecutions genuinely arising from non-political crimes or from acts contrary to the purposes and principles of the United Nations.

Article 15

1. Everyone has the right to a nationality
2. No one shall be arbitrarily deprived of his nationality nor denied the right to change his nationality.

Article 16

1. Men and women of full age, without any limitation due to race, nationality or religion, have the right to marry and to found a family. They are entitled to equal rights as to marriage, during marriage and at its dissolution.

2. Marriage shall be entered into only with the free and full consent of the intending spouses.
3. The family is the natural and fundamental group unit of society and is entitled to protection by society and the State.

Article 17

1. Everyone has the right to own property alone as well as in association with others.
2. No one shall be arbitrarily deprived of his property.

Article 18

Everyone has the right to freedom of thought, conscience and religion; this right includes freedom to change his religion or belief, and freedom, either alone or in community with others and in public or private, to manifest his religion or belief in teaching, practice, worship and observance.

Article 19

Everyone has the right to freedom of opinion and expression; this right includes freedom to hold opinions without interference and to seek, receive and impart information and ideas through any media and regardless of frontiers.

Article 20

1. Everyone has the right to freedom of peaceful assembly and association.
2. No one may be compelled to belong to an association.

Article 21

1. Everyone has the right to take part in the government of his country, directly or through freely chosen representatives.
2. Everyone has the right to equal access to public service in his country.
3. The will of the people shall be the basis of the authority of government; this will shall be expressed in periodic and genuine elections which shall be by universal and equal

suffrage and shall be held by secret vote or by equivalent free voting procedures.

Article 22

Everyone, as a member of society, has the right to social security and is entitled to realization, through national effort and international co-operation and in accordance with the organization and resources of each State, of the economic, social and cultural rights indispensable for his dignity and the free development of his personality.

Article 23

1. Everyone has the right to work, to free choice of employment, to just and favourable conditions of work and to protection against unemployment.
2. Everyone, without any discrimination, has the right to equal pay for equal work.
3. Everyone who works has the right to just and favourable remuneration ensuring for himself and his family an existence worthy of human dignity, and supplemented, if necessary, by other means of social protection.
4. Everyone has the right to form and to join trade unions for the protection of his interests.

Article 24

Everyone has the right to rest and leisure, including reasonable limitation of working hours and periodic holidays with pay.

Article 25

1. Everyone has the right to a standard of living adequate for the health and well-being of himself and of his family, including food, clothing, housing and medical care and necessary social services, and the right to security in the event of unemployment, sickness, disability, widowhood, old age or other lack of livelihood in circumstances beyond his control.
2. Motherhood and childhood are entitled to special care and assistance. All children, whether born in or out of wedlock, shall enjoy the same social protection.

Article 26

1. Everyone has the right to education. Education shall be free, at least in the elementary and fundamental stages. Elementary education shall be compulsory. Technical and professional education shall be made generally available and higher education shall be equally accessible to all on the basis of merit.
2. Education shall be directed to the full development of the human personality and to the strengthening of respect for human rights and fundamental freedoms. It shall promote understanding, tolerance and friendship among all nations, racial or religious groups, and shall further the activities of the United Nations for the maintenance of peace.
3. Parents have a prior right to choose the kind of education that shall be given to their children.

Article 27

1. Everyone has the right freely to participate in the cultural life of the community, to enjoy the arts and to share in scientific advancement and its benefits.
2. Everyone has the right to the protection of the moral and material interests resulting from any scientific, literary or artistic production of which he is the author.

Article 28

Everyone is entitled to a social and international order in which the rights and freedoms set forth in this Declaration can be fully realized.

Article 29

1. Everyone has duties to the community in which alone the free and full development of his personality is possible.
2. In the exercise of his rights and freedoms, everyone shall be subject only to such limitations as are determined by law solely for the purpose of securing due recognition and respect for the rights and freedoms of others and of meeting the just requirements of morality, public order and the general welfare in a democratic society.

3. These rights and freedoms may in no case be exercised contrary to the purposes and principles of the United Nations.

Article 30

Nothing in this Declaration may be interpreted as implying for any State, group or person any right to engage in any activity or to perform any act aimed at the destruction of any of the rights and freedoms set forth herein.

Appendix B

International Covenant on Civil and Political Rights

Preamble

The States Parties to the present Covenant,

Considering that, in accordance with the principles proclaimed in the Charter of the United Nations, recognition of the inherent dignity and of the equal and inalienable rights of all members of the human family is the foundation of freedom, justice and peace in the world.

Recognizing that these rights derive from the inherent dignity of the human person,

Recognizing that, in accordance with the Universal Declaration of Human Rights, the ideal of free human beings enjoying civil and political freedom and freedom from fear and want can only be achieved if conditions are created whereby everyone may enjoy his civil and political rights, as well as his economic, social and cultural rights,

Considering the obligation of States under the Charter of the United Nations to promote universal respect for, and observance of, human rights and freedoms,

Realizing that the individual, having duties to other individuals and to the community to which he belongs, is under a responsibility to strive for the promotion and observance of the rights recognized in the present Covenant,

Agree upon the following articles:

Part I

Article 1

1. All peoples have the right of self-determination. By virtue of that right they freely determine their political status and freely pursue their economic, social and cultural development.
2. All peoples may, for their own ends, freely dispose of their natural wealth and resources without prejudice to any obligations arising out of international economic co-operation, based upon the principle of mutual benefit, and international law. In no case may a people be deprived of its own means of subsistence.
3. The States Parties to the present Covenant, including those having responsibility for the administration of Non-Self-Governing and Trust Territories, shall promote the realization of the right of self-determination, and shall respect that right, in conformity with the provisions of the Charter of the United Nations.

Part II

Article 2

1. Each State Party to the present Covenant undertakes to respect and to ensure to all individuals within its territory and subject to its jurisdiction the rights recognized in the present Covenant, without distinction of any kind, such as race, colour, sex, language, religion, political or other opinion, national or social origin, property, birth or other status.
2. Where not already provided for by existing legislative or other measures, each State Party to the present Covenant undertakes to take the necessary steps, in accordance with its constitutional processes and with the provisions of the present Covenant, to adopt such legislative or other measures as may be necessary to give effect to the rights recognized in the present Covenant.

3. Each State Party to the present Covenant undertakes:

    (*a*) To ensure that any person whose rights or freedoms as herein recognized are violated shall have an effective remedy, notwithstanding that the violation has been committed by persons acting in an official capacity;

    (*b*) To ensure that any person claiming such a remedy shall have his right thereto determined by competent judicial, administrative or legislative authorities, or by any other competent authority provided for by the legal system of the State, and to develop the possibilities of judicial remedy;

    (*c*) To ensure that the competent authorities shall enforce such remedies when granted.

Article 3

The States Parties to the present Covenant undertake to ensure the equal right of men and women to the enjoyment of all civil and political rights set forth in the present Covenant.

Article 4

1. In time of public emergency which threatens the life of the nation and the existence of which is officially proclaimed, the States Parties to the present Covenant may take measures derogating from their obligations under the present Covenant to the extent strictly required by the exigencies of the situation, provided that such measures are not inconsistent with their other obligations under international law and do not involve discrimination solely on the ground of race, colour, sex, language, religion or social origin.

2. No derogation from articles 6, 7, 8 (paragraphs 1 and 2), 11, 15, 16 and 18 may be made under this provision.

3. Any State Party to the present Covenant availing itself of the right of derogation shall immediately inform the other States Parties to the present Covenant, through the intermediary of the Secretary-General of the United Nations, of the provisions from which it has derogated and of the reasons by which it was actuated. A further communication shall be made, through the same intermediary, on the date on which it terminates such derogation.

Article 5

1. Nothing in the present Covenant may be interpreted as implying for any State, group or person any right to engage in any activity or perform any act aimed at the destruction of any of the rights and freedoms recognized herein or at their limitation to a greater extent than is provided for in the present Covenant.

2. There shall be no restriction upon or derogation from any of the fundamental human rights recognized or existing in any State Party to the present Covenant pursuant to law, conventions, regulations or custom on the pretext that the present Covenant does not recognize such rights or that it recognizes them to a lesser extent.

Part III

Article 6

1. Every human being has the inherent right to life. This right shall be protected by law. No one shall be arbitrarily deprived of his life.

2. In countries which have not abolished the death penalty, sentence of death may be imposed only for the most serious crimes in accordance with the law in force at the time of the commission of the crime and not contrary to the provisions of the present Covenant and to the Convention on the Prevention and Punishment of the Crime of Genocide. This penalty can only be carried out pursuant to a final judgement rendered by a competent court.

3. When deprivation of life constitutes the crime of genocide, it is understood that nothing in this article shall authorize any State Party to the present Covenant to derogate in any way from any obligation assumed under the provisions of the Convention on the Prevention and Punishment of the Crime of Genocide.

4. Anyone sentenced to death shall have the right to seek pardon or commutation of the sentence. Amnesty, pardon or commutation of the sentence of death may be granted in all cases.

5. Sentence of death shall not be imposed for crimes committed by persons below eighteen years of age and shall not be carried out on pregnant women.

6. Nothing in this article shall be invoked to delay or to prevent the abolition of capital punishment by any State Party to the present Covenant.

Article 7

No one shall be subjected to torture or to cruel, inhuman or degrading treatment or punishment. In particular, no one shall be subjected without his free consent to medical or scientific experimentation.

Article 8

1. No one shall be held in slavery; slavery and the slave-trade in all their forms shall be prohibited.
2. No one shall be held in servitude.

. . .

Article 9

1. Everyone has the right to liberty and security of person. No one shall be subjected to arbitrary arrest or detention. No one shall be deprived of his liberty except on such grounds and in accordance with such procedure as are established by law.
2. Anyone who is arrested shall be informed, at the time of arrest, of the reasons for his arrest and shall be promptly informed of any charges against him.
3. Anyone arrested or detained on a criminal charge shall be brought promptly before a judge or other officer authorized by law to exercise judicial power and shall be entitled to trial within a reasonable time or to release. It shall not be the general rule that persons awaiting trial shall be detained in custody, but release may be subject to guarantees to appear for trial, at any other stage of the judicial proceedings, and, should occasion arise, for execution of the judgement.
4. Anyone who is deprived of his liberty by arrest or detention shall be entitled to take proceedings before a court, in order that court may decide without delay on the lawfulness of his detention and order his release if the detention is not lawful.
5. Anyone who has been the victim of unlawful arrest or detention shall have an enforceable right to compensation.

Article 10

1. All persons deprived of their liberty shall be treated with humanity and with respect for the inherent dignity of the human person.

2. (*a*) Accused persons shall, save in exceptional circumstances, be segregated from convicted persons and shall be subject to separate treatment appropriate to their status as unconvicted persons;

   (*b*) Accused juvenile persons shall be separated from adults and brought as speedily as possible for adjudication.

3. The penitentiary system shall comprise treatment of prisoners the essential aim of which shall be their reformation and social rehabilitation. Juvenile offenders shall be segregated from adults and be accorded treatment appropriate to their age and legal status.

Article 11

No one shall be imprisoned merely on the ground of inability to fulfil a contractual obligation.

Article 12

1. Everyone lawfully within the territory of a State shall, within that territory, have the right to liberty of movement and freedom to choose his residence.

2. Everyone shall be free to leave any country, including his own.

3. The above-mentioned rights shall not be subject to any restrictions except those which are provided by law, are necessary to protect national security, public order (*ordre public*), public health or morals or the rights and freedoms of others, and are consistent with the other rights recognized in the present Covenant.

4. No one shall be arbitrarily deprived of the right to enter his own country.

Article 13

An alien lawfully in the territory of a State Party to the present Covenant may be expelled therefrom only in pursuance of a decision reached in accordance with law and shall, except where compelling reasons of national security otherwise require, be allowed to submit the reasons against his expulsion and to have his case reviewed by, and be represented for the purpose before, the competent authority or a person or persons especially designated by the competent authority.

Article 14

1. All persons shall be equal before the courts and tribunals. In the determination of any criminal charge against him, or of his rights and obligations in a suit at law, everyone shall be entitled to a fair and public hearing by a competent, independent and impartial tribunal established by law. The press and the public may be excluded from all or part of a trial for reasons of morals, public order (*ordre public*) or national security in a democratic society, or when the interest of the private lives of the parties so requires, or to the extent strictly necessary in the opinion of the court in special circumstances where publicity would prejudice the interests of justice; but any judgement rendered in a criminal case or in a suit at law shall be made public except where the interest of juvenile persons otherwise requires or the proceedings concern matrimonial disputes or the guardianship of children.

2. Everyone charged with a criminal offence shall have the right to be presumed innocent until proved guilty according to law.

3. In the determination of any criminal charge against him, everyone shall be entitled to the following minimum guarantees, in full equality:

   (*a*) To be informed promptly and in detail in a language which he understands of the nature and cause of the charge against him;

   (*b*) To have adequate time and facilities for the preparation of his defence and to communicate with counsel of his own choosing;

   (*c*) To be tried without undue delay;

   (*d*) To be tried in his presence, and to defend himself in person or through legal assistance of his own choosing; to be informed, if he does not have legal assistance, of this right; and to have legal assistance assigned to him, in any case where the interests of justice so require, and without payment by him in any such case if he does not have sufficient means to pay for it;

(*e*) To examine, or have examined, the witnesses against him and to obtain the attendance and examination of witnesses on his behalf under the same conditions as witnesses against him;

(*f*) To have the free assistance of an interpreter if he cannot understand or speak the language used in court;

(*g*) Not to be compelled to testify against himself or to confess guilt.

4. In the case of juvenile persons, the procedure shall be such as will take account of their age and the desirability of promoting their rehabilitation.

5. Everyone convicted of a crime shall have the right to his conviction and sentence being reviewed by a higher tribunal according to law.

6. When a person has by a final decision been convicted of a criminal offence and when subsequently his conviction has been reversed or he has been pardoned on the ground that a new or newly discovered fact shows conclusively that there has been a miscarriage of justice, the person who has suffered punishment as a result of such conviction shall be compensated according to law, unless it is proved that the non-disclosure of the unknown fact in time is wholly or partly attributable to him.

7. No one shall be liable to be tried or punished again for an offence for which he has already been finally convicted or acquitted in accordance with the law and penal procedure of each country.

Article 15

1. No one shall be held guilty of any criminal offence on account of any act or omission which did not constitute a criminal offence, under national or international law, at the time when it was committed. Nor shall a heavier penalty be imposed than the one that was applicable at the time when the criminal offence was committed. If, subsequent to the commission of the offence, provision is made by law for the imposition of the lighter penalty, the offender shall benefit thereby.

2. Nothing in this article shall prejudice the trial and punishment of any person for any act or omission which, at the time when it was committed, was criminal according to the general principles of law recognized by the community of nations.

Article 16

Everyone shall have the right to recognition everywhere as a person before the law.

Article 17

1. No one shall be subjected to arbitrary or unlawful interference with his privacy, family, home or correspondence, nor to unlawful attacks on his honour and reputation.
2. Everyone has the right to the protection of the law against such interference or attacks.

Article 18

1. Everyone shall have the right to freedom of thought, conscience and religion. This right shall include freedom to have or to adopt a religion or belief of his choice, and freedom, either individually or in community with others and in public or private, to manifest his religion or belief in worship, observance, practice and teaching.
2. No one shall be subject to coercion which would impair his freedom to have or to adopt a religion or belief of his choice.
3. Freedom to manifest one's religion or beliefs may be subject only to such limitations as are prescribed by law and are necessary to protect public safety, order, health, or morals or the fundamental rights and freedoms of others.
4. The States Parties to the present Covenant undertake to have respect for the liberty of parents and, when applicable, legal guardians to ensure the religious and moral education of their children in conformity with their own convictions.

Article 19

1. Everyone shall have the right to hold opinions without interference.
2. Everyone shall have the right to freedom of expression; this right shall include freedom to seek, receive and impart information and ideas of all kinds, regardless of frontiers, either orally, in writing or in print, in the form of art, or through any other media of his choice.

3. The exercise of the rights provided for in paragraph 2 of this article carries with it special duties and responsibilities. It may therefore be subject to certain restrictions, but these shall only be such as are provided by law and are necessary:
    (*a*) For respect of the rights or reputations of others;
    (*b*) For the protection of national security or of public order (ordre public), or of public health or morals.

Article 20

1. Any propaganda for war shall be prohibited by law.
2. Any advocacy of national, racial or religious hatred that constitutes incitement to discrimination, hostility or violence shall be prohibited by law.

Article 21

The right of peaceful assembly shall be recognized. No restrictions may be placed on the exercise of this right other than those imposed in conformity with the law and which are necessary in a democratic society in the interests of national security or public safety, public order (*ordre public*), the protection of public health or morals or the protection of the rights and freedoms of others.

Article 22

1. Everyone shall have the right to freedom of association with others, including the right to form and join trade unions for the protection of his interests.
2. No restrictions may be placed on the exercise of this right other than those which are prescribed by law and which are necessary in a democratic society in the interests of national security or public safety, public order (*ordre public*), the protection of public health or morals or the protection of the rights and freedoms of others. This article shall not prevent the imposition of lawful restrictions on members of the armed forces and of the police in their exercise of this right.
    . . .

Article 23

1. The family is the natural and fundamental group unit of society and is entitled to protection by society and the State.

2. The right of men and women of marriageable age to marry and to found a family shall be recognized.
3. No marriage shall be entered into without the free and full consent of the intending spouses.
4. States Parties to the present Covenant shall take appropriate steps to ensure equality of rights and responsibilities of spouses as to marriage, during marriage and at its dissolution. In the case of dissolution, provision shall be made for the necessary protection of any children.

Article 24

1. Every child shall have, without any discrimination as to race, colour, sex, language, religion, national or social origin, property or birth, the right to such measures of protection as are required by his status as a minor, on the part of his family, society and the State.
2. Every child shall be registered immediately after birth and shall have a name.
3. Every child has the right to acquire a nationality.

Article 25

Every citizen shall have the right and the opportunity, without any of the distinctions mentioned in article 2 and without unreasonable restrictions:
(*a*) To take part in the conduct of public affairs, directly or through freely chosen representatives;
(*b*) To vote and to be elected at genuine periodic elections which shall be by universal and equal suffrage and shall be held by secret ballot, guaranteeing the free expression of the will of the electors;
(*c*) To have access, on general terms of equality, to public service in his country.

Article 26

All persons are equal before the law and are entitled without any discrimination to the equal protection of the law. In this respect, the law shall prohibit any discrimination and guarantee to all persons equal and effective protection against discrimination on any ground such as race, colour, sex, language, religion, political or other opinion, national or social origin, property, birth or other status.

Article 27

In those States in which ethnic, religious or linguistic minorities exist, persons belonging to such minorities shall not be denied the right, in community with the other members of their group, to enjoy their own culture, to profess and practise their own religion, or to use their own language.

Part IV

Article 28

1. There shall be established a Human Rights Committee (hereafter referred to in the present Covenant as the Committee). It shall consist of eighteen members and shall carry out the functions hereinafter provided.
2. The Committee shall be composed of nationals of the States Parties to the present Covenant who shall be persons of high moral character and recognized competence in the field of human rights, consideration being given to the usefulness of the participation of some persons having legal experience.
3. The members of the Committee shall be elected and shall serve in their personal capacity.

. . .

Article 31

1. The Committee may not include more than one national of the same State.
2. In the election of the Committee, consideration shall be given to equitable geographical distribution of membership and to the representation of the different forms of civilization and of the principal legal systems.

. . .

Article 38

Every member of the Committee shall, before taking up his duties, make a solemn declaration in open committee that he will perform his functions impartially and conscientiously.

. . .

Article 39

1. The Committee shall elect its officers for a term of two years. They may be re-elected.

. . .

2. (*b*) Decisions of the Committee shall be made by a majority vote of the members present.

Article 40

1. The States Parties to the present Covenant undertake to submit reports on the measures they have adopted which give effect to the rights recognized herein and on the progress made in the enjoyment of those rights:
   (*a*) Within one year of the entry into force of the present Covenant for the States Parties concerned;
   (*b*) Thereafter whenever the Committee so requests.
2. All reports shall be submitted to the Secretary-General of the United Nations, who shall transmit them to the Committee for consideration. Reports shall indicate the factors and difficulties, if any, affecting the implementation of the present Covenant.
3. The Secretary-General of the United Nations may, after consultation with the Committee, transmit to the specialized agencies concerned copies of such parts of the reports as may fall within their field of competence.
4. The Committee shall study the reports submitted by the States Parties to the present Covenant. It shall transmit its reports, and such general comments as it may consider appropriate, to the States Parties. The Committee may also transmit to the Economic and Social Council these comments along with the copies of the reports it has received from States Parties to the present Covenant.
5. The States Parties to the present Covenant may submit to the Committee observations on any comments that may be made in accordance with paragraph 4 of this article.

Article 41

1. A State Party to the present Covenant may at any time declare under this article that it recognizes the competence of the Committee to receive and consider communications to the

effect that a State Party claims that another State Party is not fulfilling its obligations under the present Covenant. Communications under this article may be received and considered only if submitted by a State Party which has made a declaration recognizing in regard to itself the competence of the Committee. No communication shall be received by the Committee if it concerns a State Party which has not made such a declaration. Communications received under this article shall be dealt with in accordance with the following procedure:

[Article 41 spells out a procedure involving efforts toward resolution, referral of the matter to the Committee, and a report by the Committee to the States Parties concerned that is confined 'to a brief statement of the facts; the written submissions and record of the oral submissions made by the States Parties concerned shall be attached to the report.' Article 42 provides that if the matter is not resolved to the satisfaction of the States Parties concerned, the Committee may, with the consent of those parties, appoint an *ad hoc* Conciliation Commission. If no amicable solution is reached, the Commission submits a report to the Chairman of the Committee. The report includes the Commission's finding on all relevant questions of fact, and its views on possibilities of an amicable solution.]

. . .

Article 44

The provisions for the implementation of the present Covenant shall apply without prejudice to the procedures prescribed in the field of human rights by or under the constituent instruments and the conventions of the United Nations and of the specialized agencies and shall not prevent the States Parties to the present Covenant from having recourse to other procedures for settling a dispute in accordance with general or special international agreements in force between them.

Article 45

The Committee shall submit to the General Assembly of the United Nations, through the Economic and Social Council, an annual report on its activities.

Part V

Article 46

Nothing in the present Covenant shall be interpreted as impairing the provisions of the Charter of the United Nations and of the constitutions of the specialized agencies which define the respective responsibilities of the various organs of the United Nations and of the specialized agencies in regard to the matters dealt with in the present Covenant.

Article 47

Nothing in the present Covenant shall be interpreted as impairing the inherent right of all peoples to enjoy and utilize fully and freely their natural wealth and resources.

Part VI

. . .

Article 50

The provisions of the present Covenant shall extend to all parts of federal States without any limitations or exceptions.

Article 51

1. Any State Party to the present Covenant may propose an amendment and file it with the Secretary-General of the United Nations. The Secretary-General of the United Nations shall thereupon communicate any proposed amendments to the States Parties to the present Covenant with a request that they notify him whether they favour a conference of States Parties for the purpose of considering and voting upon the proposals. In the event that at least one third of the States Parties favours such a conference, the Secretary-General shall convene the conference under the auspices of the United Nations. Any amendment adopted by a majority of the States Parties present and voting at the conference shall be submitted to the General Assembly of the United Nations for approval.

2. Amendments shall come into force when they have been approved by the General Assembly of the United Nations and accepted by a two-thirds majority of the States Parties to the present Covenant in accordance with their respective constitutional processes.

3. When amendments come into force, they shall be binding on those States Parties which have accepted them, other States Parties still being bound by the provisions of the present Covenant and any earlier amendment which they have accepted.

. . .

PROTOCOLS TO THE INTERNATIONAL COVENANT ON CIVIL AND POLITICAL RIGHTS

(First) Optional Protocol

The States Parties to the present Protocol,

Considering that in order further to achieve the purpose of the International Covenant on Civil and Political Rights (hereinafter referred to as the Covenant) and the implementation of its provisions it would be appropriate to enable the Human Rights Committee set up in part IV of the Covenant (hereinafter referred to as the Committee) to receive and consider, as provided in the present Protocol, communications from individuals claiming to be victims of violations of any of the rights set forth in the Covenant,

Have agreed as follows:

Article 1

A State Party to the Covenant that becomes a Party to the present Protocol recognizes the competence of the Committee to receive and consider communications from individuals subject to its jurisdiction who claim to be victims of a violation by that State Party of any of the rights set forth in the Covenant. No communication shall be received by the Committee if it concerns a State Party to the Covenant which is not a Party to the present Protocol.

Article 2

Subject to the provisions of article 1, individuals who claim that any of their rights enumerated in the Covenant have been violated and who have exhausted all available domestic remedies may submit a written communication to the Committee for consideration.

Article 3

The Committee shall consider inadmissible any communication under the present Protocol which is anonymous, or which it considers to be an abuse of the right of submission of such communications or to be incompatible with the provisions of the Covenant.

Article 4

1. Subject to the provisions of article 3, the Committee shall bring any communications submitted to it under the present Protocol to the attention of the State Party to the present Protocol alleged to be violating any provision of the Covenant.
2. Within six months, the receiving State shall submit to the Committee written explanations or statements clarifying the matter and the remedy, if any, that may have been taken by that State.

Article 5

1. The Committee shall consider communications received under the present Protocol in the light of all written information made available to it by the individual and by the State Party concerned.
2. The Committee shall not consider any communication from an individual unless it has ascertained that:
   (*a*) The same matter is not being examined under another procedure of international investigation or settlement;
   (*b*) The individual has exhausted all available domestic remedies. This shall not be the rule where the application of the remedies is unreasonably prolonged.
3. The Committee shall hold closed meetings when examining communications under the present Protocol.

4. The Committee shall forward its views to the State Party concerned and to the individual.

Article 6

The Committee shall include in its annual report under article 45 of the Covenant a summary of its activities under the present Protocol.

. . .

Second Optional Protocol

The States Parties to the present Protocol,

Believing that abolition of the death penalty contributes to enhancement of human dignity and progressive development of human rights,

Recalling article 3 of the Universal Declaration of Human Rights, adopted on 10 December 1948, and article 6 of the International Covenant on Civil and Political Rights, adopted on 16 December 1966,

Noting that article 6 of the International Covenant on Civil and Political Rights refers to abolition of the death penalty in terms that strongly suggest that abolition is desirable,

Convinced that all measures of abolition of the death penalty should be considered as progress in the enjoyment of the right to life,

Desirous to undertake hereby an international commitment to abolish the death penalty,

Have agreed as follows:

Article 1

1. No one within the jurisdiction of a State Party to the present Protocol shall be executed.
2. Each State Party shall take all necessary measures to abolish the death penalty within its jurisdiction.

Article 2

1. No reservation is admissible to the present Protocol, except for a reservation made at the time of ratification or accession that provides for the application of the death penalty in time of war pursuant to a conviction for a most serious crime of a military nature committed during wartime.

. . .

Article 3

The States Parties to the present Protocol shall include in the reports they submit to the Human Rights Committee, in accordance with article 40 of the Covenant, information on the measures that they have adopted to give effect to the present Protocol.

. . .

Appendix C

International Covenant on Economic, Social, and Cultural Rights

Preamble

The States Parties to the present Covenant,

. . .

Recognizing that these rights derive from the inherent dignity of the human person,

Recognizing that, in accordance with the Universal Declaration of Human Rights, the ideal of free human beings enjoying freedom from fear and want can only be achieved if conditions are created whereby every-one may enjoy his economic, social and cultural rights, as well as his civil and political rights,

. . .

Realizing that the individual, having duties to other individuals and to the community to which he belongs, is under a responsibility to strive for the promotion and observance of the rights recognized in the present Covenant,

Agree upon the following articles:

Part I

Article 1

1. All peoples have the right of self-determination. By virtue of that right they freely determine their political status and freely pursue their economic, social and cultural development.
2. All peoples may, for their own ends, freely dispose of their natural wealth and resources without prejudice to any obligations arising out of international economic co-operation, based upon the principle of mutual benefit, and international law. In no case may a people be deprived of its own means of subsistence.
3. The States Parties to the present Covenant, including those having responsibility for the administration of Non-Self-Governing and Trust Territories, shall promote the realization of the right of self-determination, and shall respect that right, in conformity with the provisions of the Charter of the United Nations.

Part II

Article 2

1. Each State Party to the present Covenant undertakes to take steps, individually and through international assistance and co-operation, especially economic and technical, to the maximum of its available resources, with a view to achieving progressively the full realization of the rights recognized in the present Covenant by all appropriate means, including particularly the adoption of legislative measures.
2. The States Parties to the present Covenant undertake to guarantee that the rights enunciated in the present Covenant will be exercised without discrimination of any kind as to race, colour, sex, language, religion, political or other opinion, national or social origin, property, birth or other status.
3. Developing countries, with due regard to human rights and their national economy, may determine to what extent they would guarantee the economic rights recognized in the present Covenant to non-nationals.

Article 3

The States Parties to the present Covenant undertake to ensure the equal right of men and women to the enjoyment of all economic, social and cultural rights set forth in the present Covenant.

Article 4

The States Parties to the present Covenant recognize that, in the enjoyment of those rights provided by the State in conformity with the present Covenant, the State may subject such rights only to such limitations as are determined by law only in so far as this may be compatible with the nature of these rights and solely for the purpose of promoting the general welfare in a democratic society.

Article 5

1. Nothing in the present Covenant may be interpreted as implying for any State, group or person any right to engage in any activity or to perform any act aimed at the destruction of any of the rights or freedoms recognized herein, or at their limitation to a greater extent than is provided for in the present Covenant.
2. No restriction upon or derogation from any of the fundamental human rights recognized or existing in any country in virtue of law, conventions, regulations or custom shall be admitted on the pretext that the present Covenant does not recognize such rights or that it recognizes them to a lesser extent.

Part III

Article 6

1. The States Parties to the present Covenant recognize the right to work, which includes the right of everyone to the opportunity to gain his living by work which he freely chooses or accepts, and will take appropriate steps to safeguard this right.
2. The steps to be taken by a State Party to the present Covenant to achieve the full realization of this right shall include technical and vocational guidance and training programmes, policies and

techniques to achieve steady economic, social and cultural development and full and productive employment under conditions safeguarding fundamental political and economic freedoms to the individual.

Article 7

The States Parties to the present Covenant recognize the right of everyone to the enjoyment of just and favourable conditions of work which ensure, in particular:

(a) Remuneration which provides all workers, as a minimum, with:
  (i) Fair wages and equal remuneration for work of equal value without distinction of any kind, in particular women being guaranteed conditions of work not inferior to those enjoyed by men, with equal pay for equal work;
  (ii) A decent living for themselves and their families in accordance with the provisions of the present Covenant;
(b) Safe and healthy working conditions;
(c) Equal opportunity for everyone to be promoted in his employment to an appropriate higher level, subject to no considerations other than those of seniority and competence;
(d) Rest, leisure and reasonable limitation of working hours and periodic holidays with pay, as well as remuneration for public holidays.

Article 8

1. The States Parties to the present Covenant undertake to ensure:
  (a) The right of everyone to form trade unions and join the trade union of his choice, subject only to the rules of the organization concerned, for the promotion and protection of his economic and social interests. No restrictions may be placed on the exercise of this right other than those prescribed by law and which are necessary in a democratic society in the interests of national security or public order or for the protection of the rights and freedoms of others;

(*b*) The right of trade unions to establish national federations or confederations and the right of the latter to form or join international trade-union organizations;

(*c*) The right of trade unions to function freely subject to no limitations other than those prescribed by law and which are necessary in a democratic society in the interests of national security or public order or for the protection of the rights and freedoms of others;

(*d*) The right to strike, provided that it is exercised in conformity with the laws of the particular country.

2. This article shall not prevent the imposition of lawful restrictions on the exercise of these rights by members of the armed forces or of the police or of the administration of the State.

. . .

Article 9

The States Parties to the present Covenant recognize the right of everyone to social security, including social insurance.

Article 10

The States Parties to the present Covenant recognize that:

1. The widest possible protection and assistance should be accorded to the family, which is the natural and fundamental group unit of society, particularly for its establishment and while it is responsible for the care and education of dependent children. Marriage must be entered into with the free consent of the intending spouses.

2. Special protection should be accorded to mothers during a reasonable period before and after childbirth. During such period working mothers should be accorded paid leave or leave with adequate social security benefits.

3. Special measures of protection and assistance should be taken on behalf of all children and young persons without any discrimination for reasons of parentage or other conditions. Children and young persons should be protected from economic and social exploitation. Their employment in work

harmful to their morals or health or dangerous to life or likely
to hamper their normal development should be punishable by
law. States should also set age limits below which the paid
employment of child labour should be prohibited and punishable by law.

Article 11

1. The States Parties to the present Covenant recognize the right
   of everyone to an adequate standard of living for himself and
   his family, including adequate food, clothing and housing,
   and to the continuous improvement of living conditions. The
   States Parties will take appropriate steps to ensure the realization of this right, recognizing to this effect the essential
   importance of international co-operation based on free
   consent.

2. The States Parties to the present Covenant, recognizing the
   fundamental right of everyone to be free from hunger, shall
   take, individually and through international co-operation, the
   measures, including specific programmes, which are needed:

   (*a*) To improve methods of production, conservation and
       distribution of food by making full use of technical and
       scientific knowledge, by disseminating knowledge of the
       principles of nutrition and by developing or reforming
       agrarian systems in such a way as to achieve the most
       efficient development and utilization of natural resources;

   (*b*) Taking into account the problems of both food-importing
       and food-exporting countries, to ensure an equitable
       distribution of world food supplies in relation to need.

Article 12

1. The States Parties to the present Covenant recognize the right
   of everyone to the enjoyment of the highest attainable standard
   of physical and mental health.

2. The steps to be taken by the States Parties to the present
   Covenant to achieve the full realization of this right shall
   include those necessary for:

   (*a*) The provision for the reduction of the stillbirth-rate and of
       infant mortality and for the healthy development of the child;

(*b*) The improvement of all aspects of environmental and industrial hygiene;

(*c*) The prevention, treatment and control of epidemic, endemic, occupational and other diseases;

(*d*) The creation of conditions which would assure to all medical service and medical attention in the event of sickness.

Article 13

1. The States Parties to the present Covenant recognize the right of everyone to education. They agree that education shall be directed to the full development of the human personality and the sense of its dignity, and shall strengthen the respect for human rights and fundamental freedoms. They further agree that education shall enable all persons to participate effectively in a free society, promote understanding, tolerance and friendship among all nations and all racial, ethnic or religious groups, and further the activities of the United Nations for the maintenance of peace.

2. The States Parties to the present Covenant recognize that, with a view to achieving the full realization of this right:

(*a*) Primary education shall be compulsory and available free to all;

(*b*) Secondary education in its different forms, including technical and vocational secondary education, shall be made generally available and accessible to all by every appropriate means, and in particular by the progressive introduction of free education;

(*c*) Higher education shall be made equally accessible to all, on the basis of capacity, by every appropriate means, and in particular by the progressive introduction of free education;

(*d*) Fundamental education shall be encouraged or intensified as far as possible for those persons who have not received or completed the whole period of their primary education;

(*e*) The development of a system of schools at all levels shall be actively pursued, an adequate fellowship system shall be established, and the material conditions of teaching staff shall be continuously improved.

3. The States Parties to the present Covenant undertake to have respect for the liberty of parents and, when applicable, legal guardians to choose for their children schools, other than those established by the public authorities, which conform to such minimum educational standards as may be laid down or approved by the State and to ensure the religious and moral education of their children in conformity with their own convictions.

4. No part of this article shall be construed so as to interfere with the liberty of individuals and bodies to establish and direct educational institutions, subject always to the observance of the principles set forth in paragraph I of this article and to the requirement that the education given in such institutions shall conform to such minimum standards as may be laid down by the State.

Article 14

Each State Party to the present Covenant which, at the time of becoming a Party, has not been able to secure in its metropolitan territory or other territories under its jurisdiction compulsory primary education, free of charge, undertakes, within two years, to work out and adopt a detailed plan of action for the progressive implementation, within a reasonable number of years, to be fixed in the plan, of the principle of compulsory education free of charge for all.

Article 15

1. The States Parties to the present Covenant recognize the right of everyone:
   (*a*) To take part in cultural life;
   (*b*) To enjoy the benefits of scientific progress and its applications;
   (*c*) To benefit from the protection of the moral and material interests resulting from any scientific, literary or artistic production of which he is the author.

2. The steps to be taken by the States Parties to the present Covenant to achieve the full realization of this right shall include those necessary for the conservation, the development and the diffusion of science and culture.

3. The States Parties to the present Covenant undertake to respect the freedom indispensable for scientific research and creative activity.

4. The States Parties to the present Covenant recognize the benefits to be derived from the encouragement and development of international contacts and co-operation in the scientific and cultural fields.

Part IV

Article 16

1. The States Parties to the present Covenant undertake to submit in conformity with this part of the Covenant reports on the measures which they have adopted and the progress made in achieving the observance of the rights recognized herein.

   . . .

Article 22

The Economic and Social Council may bring to the attention of other organs of the United Nations, their subsidiary organs and specialized agencies concerned with furnishing technical assistance any matters arising out of the reports referred to in this part of the present Covenant which may assist such bodies in deciding, each within its field of competence, on the advisability of international measures likely to contribute to the effective progressive implementation of the present Covenant.

Article 23

The States Parties to the present Covenant agree that international action for the achievement of the rights recognized in the present Covenant includes such methods as the conclusion of conventions, the adoption of recommendations, the furnishing of technical assistance and the holding of regional meetings and technical meetings for the purpose of consultation and study organized in conjunction with the Governments concerned.

Article 24

Nothing in the present Covenant shall be interpreted as impairing the provisions of the Charter of the United Nations and of the constitutions of the specialized agencies which define the respective responsibilities of the various organs of the United Nations and of the specialized agencies in regard to the matters dealt with in the present Covenant.

Article 25

Nothing in the present Covenant shall be interpreted as impairing the inherent right of all peoples to enjoy and utilize fully and freely their natural wealth and resources.

Part V

. . .

Article 28

The provisions of the present Covenant shall extend to all parts of federal States without any limitations or exceptions.

Appendix D

The Nuremberg Code

1. The voluntary consent of the human subject is absolutely essential.

   This means that the person involved should have legal capacity to give consent; should be so situated as to be able to exercise free power of choice, without the intervention of any element of force, fraud, deceit, duress, over-reaching, or other ulterior form of constraint or coercion; and should have sufficient knowledge and comprehension of the elements of the subject matter involved as to enable him to make an understanding and enlightened decision. This latter element requires that before the acceptance of an affirmative decision by the experimental subject there should be made known to him the nature, duration, and purpose of the experiment; the method and means by which it is to be conducted; all inconveniences and hazards reasonably to be expected; and the effects upon his health or person, which may possibly come from his participation in the experiment.

   The duty and responsibility for ascertaining the quality of the consent rests upon each individual who initiates, directs or engages in the experiment. It is a personal duty and responsibility which may not be delegated to another with impunity.

2. The experiment should be such as to yield fruitful results for the good of society, unprocurable by other methods or means of study, and not random and unnecessary in nature.

3. The experiment should be so designed and based on the results of animal experimentation and a knowledge of the natural history of the disease or other problem under study that the anticipated results will justify the performance of the experiment.

4. The experiment should be so conducted as to avoid all unnecessary physical and mental suffering and injury.

5. No experiment should be conducted where there is an *a priori* reason to believe that death or disabling injury will occur; except, perhaps, in those experiments where the experimental physicians also serve as subjects.

6. The degree of risk to be taken should never exceed that determined by the humanitarian importance of the problem to be solved by the experiment.

7. Proper preparations should be made and adequate facilities provided to protect the experimental subject against even remote possibilities of injury, disability, or death.

8. The experiment should be conducted only by scientifically qualified persons. The highest degree of skill and care should be required through all stages of the experiment of those who conduct or engage in the experiment.

9. During the course of the experiment the human subject should be at liberty to bring the experiment to an end if he has reached the physical or mental state where continuation of the experiment seemed to him to be impossible.

10. During the course of the experiment the scientist in charge must be prepared to terminate the experiment at any stage, if he has probable cause to believe, in the exercise of the good faith, superior skill, and careful judgement required of him, that a continuation of the experiment is likely to result in injury, disability, or death to the experimental subject.

Notes

Chapter 1

1. This chapter is adapted from Annas, G. J., Terrorism and Human Rights (in) Jonathan D. Moreno, ed., *In the Wake of Terror: Medicine and Morality in the Time of Crisis*, Cambridge, Mass.: MIT Press, 2003, 33–49.

2. Annas, G. J., Our Most Important Product (in) *Some Choice: Law, Medicine, and the Market*, New York: Oxford University Press, 1998, 140–152.

3. Mark Bowden, *Black Hawk Down*, New York: Penguin Books, 2000, 345–346 (emphasis in original).

4. Morgenstern, J., War is Hell, Effects Sell: *We Were Soldiers* Loses Message in the Shelling, *Wall Street Journal*, March 1, 2002, W1, W4. Morgenstern concluded his review, "Those who think such films will strengthen Americans' resolve in the war on terrorism, or any other, aren't watching the big picture on the screen."

5. J. R. R. Tolkien, *The Lord of the Rings*, New York: Ballantine Books, 1954, 82. On the one-year anniversary of the invasion of Iraq, March 19, 2004, President Bush continued to paint the world in black-and-white, good-versus-evil terms: "There is no neutral ground—no neutral ground—in the fight between civilization and terror, because there is no neutral ground between good and evil, freedom and slavery and life and death." Stevenson, R. W., President, Marking Anniversary of War, Urges World to Unite to Combat Terrorism, *New York Times*, March 20, 2004, A7.

6. Caplan, A., New World Calls for New Health Care, September 28, 2001, MSNBC.

7. Gostin, L., et al., Model State Emergency Health Powers Act, originally posted on the Internet (but since removed) October 23, 2001 (text is available from the author).

8. Seelye, K. Q., A P.O.W. Tangle: What the Law Says, *New York Times*, January 29, 2002, A14.

9. International Committee of the Red Cross, *The Geneva Conventions of August 12, 1949*, ICRC: Geneva, 1949, 81.

10. Sennott, C., and Bender, B., US Handling of War Captives Draws Fire, *Boston Globe*, January 23, 2002, A1, A10.

11. Seelye, K., and Sanger, D., Bush Reconsiders His Stand on Status of the Detainees, *New York Times*, January 29, 2002, A1, A14.

12. Seelye, K. Q., In Shift, Bush Says Geneva Rules Fit Taliban Captives, *New York Times*, February 8, 2002, 1. On June 28, 2004, the U.S. Supreme Court ruled that the U.S. Constitution requires that U.S. courts have jurisdiction over the prisoners at Guantanamo. The Court found it unnecessary to reach the question of the Geneva Conventions. *Rasul v. Bush*, 2004 LEXIS 4760.

13. Burns, J. F., After Battle, Injured Foes Are Treated with Allies, *New York Times*, March 10, 2002, 18.

14. Darraj, S. M., Model Legislation: Balancing Civil Rights and Public Health, *Johns Hopkins Public Health Magazine*, Fall 2001, available at http://www.jhsph.edu/magazine/model.htm.

15. Karl Von Clausewitz, *On War*, Washington, D.C.: Infantry Journal Press, 1950, 51.

16. Copeland, L., CDC Proposes Bioterrorism Laws, *USA Today*, November 8, 2001, 3A.

17. Supra note 14.

18. "The language and content of this draft Model State Emergency Health Powers Act do not represent the official policy, endorsement, or views of the Center for Law and the Public's Health, the CDC, NGA, NCSL, ASTHO, NACCHO, or NAAG, or other governmental or private agencies, departments, institutions, or organizations which have provided funding or guidance to the Center for Law and the Public's Health. This draft is prepared to facilitate and encourage communication among the various interested parties and stakeholders about the complex issues pertaining to the use of state emergency health powers."

Gostin, L., et al., Model State Emergency Health Powers Act, http://www.publichealthlaw.net, December 21, 2001. To underline the point that the act was not endorsed by anyone, including its financial sponsor, the director of the CDC, Jeffrey Koplan, responded to a letter written by the New England Coalition for Law and Public Health. In his words, "The draft model act does not represent any official or unofficial CDC position."

19. Mariner, W., Bioterrorism Act: The Wrong Response, *National Law Journal*, December 17, 2001.

20. Supra note 14. *See* Annas, G. J., Blinded by Bioterrorism: Public Health and Liberty in the 21st Century, *Health Matrix* 2003; 13: 33–70.

21. José Saramago, *Blindness*, New York: Harcourt (Giovanni Pontiero, tr.), 1997, 222.

22. Mishra, R., and Daley, B., New Bill Targets Disease, *Boston Globe*, November 11, 2001, B1, B7.

23. Barbera, J., et al., Large-Scale Quarantine Following Biological Terrorism in the United States: Scientific Examination, Logistic and Legal Limits, and Possible Consequences, *JAMA* 2001; 286: 2711–2717.

24. Annas, G. J., Where Are the Health Lawyers When We Need Them? *Medicolegal News* 1978; 6.2: 3, 25. *See also* Annas, G. J., Bioterrorism, Public Health, and Civil Liberties, *New England Journal of Medicine* 2002; 346: 1337–1342.

25. The most supportive organization, the National Conference of State Legislatures, set forth its views in June 2002: "NCSL does not endorse or recommend passage of the Model State Emergency Powers Act. This document [the Act] and the checklist questions are provided as a service to legislators and their staff who are considering changes to state statutes regarding public health emergencies." Lisa Speissegger and Cheryl Runyon, *The Model State Emergency Health Powers Act: A Checklist of Issues*, Washington, D.C.: NCSL, 2002, 1.

26. *See* Annas, G. J., supra note 20, at 64–66. *See also* Board of Global Health, Forum on Microbial Threats, Institute of Medicine, *Learning from SARS: Preparing for the Next Disease Outbreak (Workshop Summary)*, Washington, D.C.: National Academies Press, 2004, and Heymann, D. L., and Rodier, G., Global Surveillance, National Surveillance, and SARS, *Emerging Infectious Diseases* 2004; 10(2): 173–175.

27. Gerberding, J., et al., Bioterrorism Preparedness and Response: Clinicians and Public Health Agencies as Essential Partners, *JAMA* 2002; 287: 898–900.

28. Connolly, C., Vaccine Plan Revives Doubts on Anthrax Policy, *Washington Post*, December 24, 2001, A1.

29. Food and Drug Administration, New Drug and Biological Products: Evidence Needed to Demonstrate Efficacy of New Drugs for Use Against Lethal or Permanently Disabling Toxic Substances When Efficacy Studies in Humans Cannot be Conducted, *Federal Register* 1999; 64: 53, 960 et seq.

30. Annas, G. J., Protecting Soldiers from Friendly Fire: The Consent Requirement for Using Investigational Drugs and Vaccines in Combat, *American Journal of Law and Medicine* 1998; 24: 245–259; Food and Drug Administration, Supplementary Information on Interim Final Rule: Human Drugs and Biologics, Determination that Informed Consent Is NOT Feasible or Is Contrary to the Interests of Recipients—Revocation of 1990 Interim Final Rule and Establishment of New Interim Final Rule, *Federal Register* 1999; 64: 54, 180 et seq. These new rules were used in the Iraq war. McNeil, D. G., Drug Tested in Gulf War Is Approved for Troops, *New York Times*, February 6, 2003, A19. This approval was not without controversy. Cohen, J., New Rule Triggers Debate over Best Way to Test Drugs, *Science* 2003; 200: 1651.

31. Smallpox Vaccination Plan, Hearing Before Senate Appropriations Committee, Subcommittee on Labor, Health and Human Services, and Education, 108th Congress (2003), Statement of Julie L. Gerberding, Director, Centers for Disease Control and Prevention, available at www.lexis.com.

32. *See generally* Annas, G. J., Puppy Love: Bioterrorism, Civil Rights, and Public Health, *Florida Law Review* 2003; 1171, 1176–1177. *See also* McNeil, D. G., Two Programs to Vaccinate for Smallpox Come to a Halt, *New York Times*, June 19, 2003, A13, and Stevenson, R. W. and Stolberg, S. G., Bush Lays Out Plan on Smallpox Shots: Military Is First, *New York Times*, December 14, 2002, Al.

33. Horton, R., Public Health: A Neglected Counterterrorist Measure, *Lancet* 2001; 358: 1112–1113. On the two-year anniversary of 9/11, Robert Wright made a similar point in a long Op-ed in the *New York Times*:

> One can imagine national and global policing regimes that could keep us fairly secure even then [after an American city has been destroyed by terrorists], but they would be severe, with expanded monitoring of everyday life and shrinking civil liberties. In other words, the age-old tradeoff between security and liberty increasingly involves a third variable: antipathy. The less hatred there is in the world, the more security we can have without sacrificing personal freedom. Assuming we like our liberty, we have little choice but to take an earnest interest in the situation of distant and seemingly strange people, working to elevate their welfare, exploring their discontent as a step toward expanding their moral horizons, and in the process expanding ours. Global governance without global moral progress could be very unpleasant.

Wright, R., Two Years Later, a Thousand Years Ago, *New York Times*, September 11, 2003, A27.

34. Amartya Sen, *Development as Freedom*, New York: Anchor Books, 1999, 53.

35. *Terminiello v. Chicago*, 337 U.S. 1 (1949) (Jackson, dissenting).

36. Opening Speeches of Chief Prosecutors, *The Trial of German Major War Criminals*, vol. 1, London: His Majesty's Stationery Office, 1946, 5.

Chapter 2

1. This chapter is adapted from Annas, G. J., Human Rights and Health— The Universal Declaration of Human Rights at 50, *New England Journal of Medicine* 1998; 339: 1778–1781.

2. Knox, B., Introduction (in) Sophocles, *The Three Theban Plays: Antigone, Oedipus the King, Oedipus at Colonus*, New York: Viking Penguin, 1984.

3. M. Cherif Bassiouni, *Crimes Against Humanity in International Criminal Law*, Dordrecht, The Netherlands: Martinus Nijhoff, 1992.

4. Henry J. Steiner and Philip Alston, *International Human Rights in Context: Law, Politics, Morals*, 2nd ed., New York: Oxford University Press, 2000.

5. Steiner, H. J., Securing Human Rights: The First Half-Century of the Universal Declaration, and Beyond, *Harvard Magazine* 1998; Sept.–Oct.: 45–46.

6. Kunz, J., The United Nations Declaration of Human Rights, *American Journal of International Law* 1949; 43: 316–322.

7. Palmer, J., Hollow Celebration of 50 Years of Human-Rights Campaigning, *Lancet* 1998; 351: 1940.

8. Supra note 6.

9. Benatar, S. R., Global Disparities in Health and Human Rights: A Critical Commentary, *American Journal of Public Health* 1998; 88: 295–300.

10. Somerville, M. A., Making Health, Not War: Musings on Global Disparities in Health and Human Rights, *American Journal of Public Health* 1998; 88: 301–303.

11. Kofi Annan's Astonishing Facts!, *New York Times*, September 27, 1998, 16 wk.

12. World Bank, *World Development Report, 1993: Investing in Health*, New York: Oxford University Press, 1993.

13. World Bank, *Breaking the Conflict Trap: Civil War and Development Policy*, Geneva: World Bank, 2003. *See also* editorial, A More Challenging Summit than Everest, *Lancet* 2003; 361: 1837.

14. Mann, J., Human Rights and AIDS: The Future of the Pandemic, *John Marshall Law Review* 1996; 30: 195–206.

15. Stephenson, J., International AIDS Conference Faces "New Realism" of Advances, Obstacles, *JAMA* 1998; 280: 587–589; Donnelly, J., More Cash, Challenges in HIV Fight, Nations Viewed as Unprepared to Help Patients, *Boston Globe*, May 19, 2003, A1.

16. Robert Beaglehole and Ruth Bonita, *Public Health at the Crossroads*, Cambridge: Cambridge University Press, 1997; Mann, J., Medicine and Public Health, Ethics and Human Rights, *Hastings Center Report* 1997; 227(6): 6–13.

17. *Compare* the following by Jonathan Mann: ". . . Since 1990 all graduates of the Harvard School of Public Health receive two scrolls at commencement. The first is the degree they have earned. The second is a copy of the Universal Declaration of Human Rights, their common birthright. The dean reminds graduates that the Universal Declaration of Human Rights is as vital to their future in public health as the Hippocratic Oath or similar document would be to a medical doctor. In this way, we symbolize the inherent rich, complex, difficult, and ultimately indispensable linkage between society and health, for which we in public health have a special role and responsibility." Supra note 14.

18. This is a trend I discussed in detail in my book *Standard of Care: The Law of American Bioethics*, New York: Oxford University Press, 1993. *See also* Grodin, M., and Annas, G. J., Legacies of Nuremberg, *JAMA* 1996; 276: 1682–1683.

19. Pauline Maier, *American Scripture: Making the Declaration of Independence*, New York: Knopf, 1997.

20. Garry Wills, *Lincoln at Gettysburg: The Words that Remade America*, New York: Simon & Schuster, 1992.

Chapter 3

1. This chapter is adapted from Annas, G. J., The Man on the Moon, Immortality, and Other Millennial Myths: The Prospects and Perils of Human Genetic Engineering, *Emory Law Journal* 2000; 49: 753–782, which should be consulted for more detailed references.

2. Jonathan Riley-Smith, ed., *The Oxford Illustrated History of the Crusades*, Oxford: Oxford University Press, 1995.

3. Samuel Eliot Morison, *Admiral of the Ocean Sea: A Life of Christopher Columbus*, Boston: Little, Brown, 1942, 229.

4. Kirkpatrick Sale, *The Conquest of Paradise; Christopher Columbus and the Columbian Legacy*, New York: Knopf, 1991, 93; *see also* Hugh Thomas, *Conquest: Montezuma, Cortés, and the Fall of Old Mexico*, New York: Simon & Schuster, 1993, 156.

5. *See, e.g.*, Roberts, L., Disease and Death in the New World, *Science* 1989; 246: 1245.

6. William H. Prescott, *The History of the Conquest of Mexico*, 1843; Chicago: University of Chicago Press, 1966, 136, 370. It is an eerie coincidence of history that the map of the Aztec capital, Tenochtitlan, was first published in Nuremberg, Germany (in 1524), Thomas, supra note 4, at 268.

7. *See, e.g.*, Linda Hutcheon, *The Politics of Postmodernism,* 2nd ed., New York: Routledge, 2002.

8. *See generally* Steiner and Alston, supra note 4, Chapter 2.

9. Paul Fussell, *Wartime*, New York: Oxford University Press, 1989, 117.

10. *See generally* George J. Annas and Michael Grodin, eds., *The Nazi Doctors and the Nuremberg Code: Human Rights in Human Experimentation*, New York: Oxford University Press, 1993.

11. See Robert Proctor, *Racial Hygiene: Medicine Under the Nazis*, Cambridge, Mass: Harvard University Press, 1988.

12. *Ibid. See also* Proctor, R., Nazi Doctors, Racial Medicine, and Human Experimentation (in) *The Nazi Doctors*, supra note 10 at 17–31, and Daniel Keveles, *In the Name of Eugenics*, New York: Knopf, 1985.

13. These three documents are reprinted in Appendixes A, B, and C.

14. Walter McDougall, *The Heavens and the Earth: A Political History of the Space Age*, New York: Basic Books, 1985.

15. Norman Mailer, *Of a Fire on the Moon*, New York: New American Library, 1969.

16. *Ibid.* at 337.

17. Keller, B., Nyet: How the Soviets Lost the Race to the Moon, *New York Times Magazine,* June 27, 1990, 30, 63.

18. Supra note 14, at 413.

19. Jorge Luis Borges, The Immortals (in) *The Aleph and Other Stories, 1933–69*, New York: E. P. Dutton (di Giovanni, tr.), 1978, 165–179

20. Arthur Clarke, *2001: A Space Odyssey*, New York: New American Library, 1993.

21. Quoted in Jaroff, L., The Gene Hunt, *Time*, March 20, 1989, 63, 67.

22. *See generally* Robert J. Lifton, *The Future of Immortality and Other Essays for a Nuclear Age*, New York: Basic Books, 1987.

23. Quoted in Fisher, L. M., The Race to Cash in on the Genetic Code, *New York Times*, August 29, 1999, 3: 1. *See also* Callahan, Death and the Research Imperative, *New England Journal of Medicine* 2000; 342: 654–655.

24. Wilmut, I., et al., Viable Offspring Derived from Fetal and Adult Mammalian Cells, *Nature* 1997; 385: 810.

25. *E.g.*, Ian Wilmut, Keith Campbell, and Colin Tudge, *The Second Creation: Dolly and the Age of Biological Control*, New York: Farrar, Straus & Giroux, 2000.

26. *See* Annas, G. J., Human Cloning: A Choice or an Echo? *Dayton Law Review* 1998; 23: 256–257; and Varmus, H., Lost Your Little Boy? We'll Make Another, *New York Times*, May 2, 2004, AR 18.

27. Ya-Ping, T., et al., Genetic Enhancement of Learning and Memory in Mice, *Nature* 1999; 401: 63.

28. Quoted in Wade, N., The Hidden Traps in Fooling Mother Nature, *New York Times*, September 5, 1999, sec. 4, 1.

29. Leon Kass has been making this point for some time. *See, e.g., Toward a More Natural Science*, New York: Free Press, 1985.

30. *See, e.g.,* Elie Wiesel, *Night*, New York: MacGibbon & Kee, 1960.

31. *See generally* Georges Canguilhem, *The Normal and the Pathological*, Cambridge, Mass.: MIT Press, 1994 (translation by C. R. Fawcett of a 1963 addition to the 1943 book).

32. Kass, L., The Moral Meaning of Genetic Technology, *Commentary*, September 1999, 32, 38. *See also* Stephen S. Hall, *Merchants of Immortality: Chasing the Dream of Human Life Extension*, Boston: Houghton Mifflin, 2003.

33. *See, e.g.,* Renée Fox and Judith Swazey, *Spare Parts*, New York: Oxford University Press, 1992.

34. Olaf Stapledon imagined many possible changes in the human species in his *Last and First Man*, New York: Dover Publications, 1931.

35. Katherine Dunn explores this in her novel *Geek Love*, New York: Knopf, 1989, in which Aloysius Binewski, a carnival owner, exposes his wife to a variety of teratogens to produce children suitable for carnival acts.

36. Sven Lindqvist, *Exterminate All the Brutes*, New York: New Press, 1992. "[D]uring nineteenth-century European expansion . . . genocide began to be regarded as an inevitable by-product of progress," 122–123. *See also* Adam Hochschild, *King Leopold's Ghost*, Boston: Houghton Mifflin, 1998.

37. *See, e.g.*, Elizabeth Haiken, *Venus Envy: A History of Cosmetic Surgery*, Baltimore: Johns Hopkins University Press, 1997, and Green, M., and Lipton, M. A., Beautiful Dreamers, *People*, June 7, 2004, 58.

38. *E.g.,* "Reprogenetics" cheerleader Lee Silver suggests that the genetically enriched will develop into a separate, superior, species. *Remaking Eden*, New York: Avon, 1997.

39. H. G. Wells, *The Complete Short Stories of H. G. Wells. See also* Stapledon, supra note 34.

40. H. G. Wells, *The Time Machine*, New York: TOR, 1992 (originally published in 1895).

41. Robert Proctor, *The Nazi War on Cancer*, Princeton, N.J.: Princeton University Press, 1999, 278.

42. Michael Crichton, *Jurassic Park*, New York: Alfred A. Knopf, 1990, x.

43. Havel, V., Paying Back the West, *New York Review of Books*, September 23, 1999, 54.

44. I proposed a moratorium on human gene transfer experiments in early February 2000 in response to a question posed by science reporter Michael

Lasalandra of the *Boston Herald*. Lasalandra, M., Medical Ethicist Says Halt Gene Therapy, *Boston Herald*, February 8, 2000, 18. Later, at Asilomar, David Baltimore, a leading advocate of genetic research, is quoted as having said that it is "absolutely necessary" for gene therapists to slow down and reexamine the standards for when to begin trials on human subjects. "There are times when things shouldn't happen [gene vectors] . . . that weren't working in animals are going into humans. A lot of us are saying what the hell are [doctors] doing putting these into people?" Quoted in Barinaga, M., Asilomar Revisted: Lessons for Today? *Science* 2000; 287: 1584, 1585.

The confusion between treatment and research (gene therapy and gene transfer experiments) continues to elude many researchers, who even in light of deaths and induced cancers continue to insist that this technology should be judged "like any other treatment" in which "a fair assessment of the risk/benefit ratio should really be the only ethical criterion underlying the decision to use it." Cavazzana-Calvo, M., Thrasher, A., and Mavilio, F., The Future of Gene Therapy: Balancing the Risks and Benefits of Clinical Trials, *Nature* 2004; 427: 779–781. However, because of their inherent danger and uniqueness, special regulatory oversight is justified, and no ethical shortcuts should be taken just to placate potential investors. Moreover, insofar as the authors are correct in asserting that the risk/benefit assessment is the key ethical issue (even if not the only one), this assessment should ultimately be made by the research subject him or herself—meaning that children should not be used as subjects for gene transfer experiments until they are proven safe in adults. *See also* Caplan, A., Is Biomedical Research Too Dangerous to Pursue? *Science* 2004; 303: 1142.

45. I have never found either line particularly meaningful or useful. *See, e.g.,* Elias, S., and Annas, G. J., Somatic and Germline Gene Therapy (in) George J. Annas and Sherman Elias, eds., *Gene Mapping: Using Law and Ethics as Guides*, New York: Oxford University Press, 1993, 142–154.

46. *See also* Joy, B., Why the Future Doesn't Need Us, *Wired*, April, 2000, 238. Joy argues that it is past time for humanity to be concerned that developments in robotics, genetic engineering, and nanotechnology could create self-replicating, uncontrollable creatures that could destroy humanity.

47. Carolyn Raffensperger and Joel A. Tickner, eds., *Protecting Public Health and the Environment: Implementing the Precautionary Principle*, Washington, D.C.: Island Press, 1999. *See also* Andorno, R., The Precautionary Principle: A New Legal Standard for a Technological Age, *Journal of International Biotechnology Law* 2004; 1: 11–19. I used to separate species-altering and species-endangering activities into two categories, but I now think it makes more conceptual sense to use species-endangering as the category, and to see some forms of species-altering procedures as a subcategory of species-endangering activities.

48. Alan Shepard and Deke Slayton, *Moon Shot: The Inside Story of America's Race to the Moon*, Atlanta: Turner Publishing, 1994, 23. Aldrin never really recovered from being the second, rather than the first, man on the moon, and being first remains an American obsession. *See* Susan Faludi, *Stiffed: The Betrayal of the American Man*, New York: William Morrow, 1999, 451–468.

Chapter 4

1. This chapter is adapted from Annas, G. J., Andrews, L. B., and Isasi, R. M., Protecting the Endangered Human: Toward an International Treaty Prohibiting Cloning and Inheritable Alterations, *American Journal of Law & Medicine* 2002; 28: 151–178, which contains more detailed notes and references, and Annas, G. J., Cell Division, *Boston Globe*, April 21, 2002, D1.

2. M. Cherif Bassiouni, supra note 3, Chapter 2.

3. *See, e.g.*, Francis Fukuyama, *Our Posthuman Future*, New York: Farrar, Straus & Giroux, 2002.

4. *See, e.g.*, Raffensperger and Tickner, supra note 47, Chapter 3.

5. This proposed convention is the product of many people, including the participants at a September 21–22, 2001, conference at Boston University, Beyond Cloning: Protecting Humanity from Species-Altering Procedures. The treaty language was the subject of a roundtable that concluded the conference. The authors, together with others, most especially Patricia Baird and Alexander Capron, had drafted language to be considered at the conference and revised it after the conference based on the discussion that occurred there. The original draft also included a codicil to encourage individual countries to examine broader issues related to the regulation of assisted human reproduction and a prohibition on the patenting of human genes.

6. National Bioethics Advisory Commission, *Cloning Human Beings*, Bethesda, Md.: NBAC, 1997. *See also* President's Council on Bioethics, *Human Cloning and Human Dignity*, New York: Public Affairs, 2002, which recommends banning human reproductive cloning and placing a time-limited moratorium on research cloning.

7. National Research Council, *Scientific and Medical Aspects of Human Reproductive Cloning*, Washington, D.C.: National Academy Press, 2002. "Human reproductive cloning . . . is dangerous and likely to fail. The panel therefore unanimously supports the proposal that there should be a legally enforceable ban on the practice of human reproductive cloning. . . . The scientific and medical considerations related to this ban should be reviewed within 5 years. The ban should be reconsidered only if at least two conditions are met: (1) a new scientific and medical review indicates that the procedures are likely to be safe and effective and (2) a broad national dialogue on the societal, religious, and ethical issues suggests that a reconsideration of the ban is warranted" (at ES-1). *See also* National Research Council, *Stem Cells and the Future of Regenerative Medicine*, Washington, D.C.: National Academy Press, 2001; and Jaenisch, R., and Wilmut, I., Don't Clone Humans!, *Science* 2001; 291: 2552. "We believe attempts to clone human beings at a time when the scientific issues of nuclear cloning have not been clarified are dangerous and irresponsible." *And see* infra note 27.

8. Stuart A. Newman, oral presentation at the Beyond Cloning conference, Boston University, Boston, September 21, 2001. Other scientists have concluded that nuclear transfer cloning in primates, including humans, is simply "unachievable" with "current approaches." Simerly, C., et al., Molecular Correlates of Primate Nuclear Failures, *Science* 2003; 300: 297.

9. *See, e.g.*, Gordon, J. W., Genetic Enhancement in Humans, *Science* 1999; 283: 202–203.

10. Hans Jonas, for example, argued that is a crime against the clone to deprive the cloned child of his or her "existential right to certain subjective terms of being . . . the right to ignorance [of facts about the original that are likely to be] paralyzing for the spontaneity of becoming himself . . . in brief, the clone is antecedently robbed of the freedom which only under the protection of ignorance can thrive: and to rob a human-to-be of that freedom deliberately is an inexplicable crime that must not be committed even once." Hans Jonas, *Philosophical Essays: From Ancient Creed to Technological Man*, New York: Prentice Hall, 1974, 162–163. *See also* Jurgen Habermas, *The Future of Human Nature*, Cambridge, U.K.: Polity Press, 2003, 53–66.

11. Adams, T., Interview: The Clone Arranger, *The Observer* (*London*), December 2, 2001, 3. *See also* Winston, R., The Promise of Cloning for Human Medicine, *British Medical Journal* 1997; 314: 913–914 (arguing in favor of using cloning to help infertile men have genetically related children).

12. *See generally* Shapiro, M. H., I Want a Girl (Boy) Just Like the Girl (Boy) That Married Dear Old Dad (Mom): Cloning Lives, *Southern California Interdisciplinary Law Journal* 1999; 9: 1.

13. *E.g.*, American Society of Reproductive Medicine, Ethics Committee, Human Somatic Cell Nuclear Transfer (Cloning), November, 2000, available at http://www.asrm.org/Media/Ethics/cloning.pdf.

14. Robertson, J., Two Models of Human Cloning, *Hofstra Law Review* 1999; 27: 609.

15. Ronald Dworkin, *Sovereign Virtue: The Theory and Practice of Equality*, Cambridge, Mass.: Harvard University Press, 2000, 437–442.

16. Leon R. Kass, *Toward a More Natural Science: Biology and Human Affairs*, New York: Free Press, 1985, 110–111.

17. Rael, *The True Face of God*, Geneva: International Raelian Movement, 1998. *See generally* Stephen S. Hall, *Merchants of Immortality*, New York: Houghton Mifflin, 2003.

18. Lee Silver, *Remaking Eden: Cloning and Beyond in a Brave New World*, New York: Avon Books, 1997.

19. Pinker, S., Better Babies? Why Genetic Enhancement Is Too Unlikely to Worry About, *Boston Globe*, June 1, 2003, D1.

20. Rosario Isasi has compiled all of the national legislation related to cloning and human genetic engineering. It appears on the Global Lawyers and Physicians Web site, www.glphr.org.

21. *See* Annas and Grodin, supra note 10, Chapter 3.

22. Jonas, supra note 10.

23. It is in this sense that children become "manufactured" products. *See* Kass, supra note 16.

24. *See* Fukuyama, supra note 3, and Maxwell Mehlman, *Wondergenes*, Bloomington: University of Indiana Press, 2003, 183–191. *But see* Gregory Stock and John Campbell, eds., *Engineering the Human Germline*, New York: Oxford University Press, 2000, for arguments favoring germline engineering.

25. *See, e.g.*, the post-Dolly experiments designed to use cloning techniques to make "better animals," which was always Ian Wilmut and Keith Campbell's plan for cloning technology. *And see* Annas, G. J., Genism, Racism, and the Prospect of Genetic Genocide, *Pacific Ecologist* Spring 2003: 43–45. Shnieke, A. E., et al., Human Factor IX Trans-genic Sheep Produced by Transfer of Nuclei from Transplanted Fetal Fibroblasts, *Science* 1997; 278: 2130. On enhancement generally, *see* Sheila Rothman and David Rothman, *The Pursuit of Perfection*, New York: Pantheon Books, 2003.

26. *See* Kress's Beggars series, *Beggars in Spain*, New York: Avon, 1993; *Beggars and Choosers*, New York: Tom Doherty, 1994; and *Beggars Ride*, New York: Tom Doherty, 1996.

27. "Regulatory arbitrage" is a fancy term for seeking overseas venues to avoid local research regulations. Until early 2004, one such venue was South Korea, where there had been no laws forbidding either research or reproductive cloning. The announcement by Korean researchers in February 2004 that they had derived an embryonic stem cell from a human embryo created by somatic cell nuclear transfer (Hwang, W. S., et al., Evidence of a Pluripotent Human Embryonic Stem Cell Line Derived from a Cloned Blastocyst, *Science* 2004; 303: 1669), however, led the South Korean government to suspend their work pending the development of national regulations. Hwang initially said, "If Korea were to prohibit therapeutic cloning, we would go to other countries where it is permitted—Singapore, mainland China, maybe Great Britain. But my hope is that the Korean government will give us the license to do this kind of research. If they don't, we will move." Dreifus, C., 2 Friends, 242 Eggs and a Breakthrough, *New York Times*, February 17, 2004, D1. Two weeks later, however, he had suspended his work and was waiting for his government to decide if he could resume it, saying that he wanted such ethical guidelines and that he and his team had agreed not to transfer the cloning technology overseas without the government's permission. Faiola, A., Dr. Clone: Creating Life or Trying to Save It?, *Washington Post*, February 29, 2004. Reproductive cloning remains irresponsible. *See* Hall, S., Spector of Cloning May Prove a Mirage, *New York Times*, February 17, 2004, D1.

28. In 2004 the President's Council on Bioethics published its *Reproduction and Responsibility: The Regulation of the New Biotechnologies*, which made a set of legislative recommendations to Congress, the most significant of which are to:

> Prohibit attempts to conceive a child by any means other than the union of egg and sperm.
> Prohibit attempts to conceive a child by using gametes obtained from a human fetus or derived from human embryonic stem cells.
> Prohibit attempts to conceive a child by fusing blastomeres from two or more embryos.
> Prohibit the use of human embryos in research beyond a designated stage in their development (between 10 and 14 days after fertilization).
> Prohibit the buying and selling of human embryos. (at 222–223)

Some Council members believed that the "prohibit attempts to conceive a child" language would prove superior to "prohibit attempts to initiate a pregnancy" language and so break the current congressional deadlock on cloning legislation. This would be welcome, but seems unlikely.

29. Thucydides, *History of the Peloponnesian War*, London: Penguin Books, 1954 (Rex Warner, tr.), 147.

30. *Id.* at 242.

Chapter 5

1. This chapter was originally published as Annas, G. J., The Right to Health and the Nevirapine Case in South Africa, *New England Journal of Medicine* 2003; 348: 750–754.

2. McGreal, C., The Shame of the New South Africa, *The Guardian (London)*, November 1, 2002, 2.

3. Jonathan M. Mann, Sofia Gruskin, Michael A. Grodin, and George J. Annas, eds., *Health and Human Rights: A Reader*, New York: Routledge, 1999, 216–226.

4. Farmer, P., The Major Infectious Disease in the World: To Treat or Not to Treat? *New England Journal of Medicine* 2001; 345: 208–210.

5. Makgoba, M. W., HIV/AIDS: The Peril of Pseudoscience, *Science* 2000; 288: 1171.

6. Swarns, R. L., An AIDS Skeptic in South Africa Feeds Simmering Doubts, *New York Times*, March 31, 2002, 4.

7. Editorial, South Africa's Moral Victory, *Lancet* 2001; 357: 1303.

8. Guay, L. A., Musoke, P., Fleming, T., et al., Intrapartum and Neonatal Single-Dose Nevirapine Compared with Zidovudine for Prevention of Mother-to-Child Transmission of HIV-1 in Kampala, Uganda: HIVNET 012 Randomized Trial, *Lancet* 1999; 354: 795–802.

9. *Treatment Action Campaign v. Minister of Health*, High Court of South Africa, Transvaal Provincial Division, 2002(4) BCLR 356(T) (December 12, 2001).

10. *Minister of Health v. Treatment Action Campaign*, Constitutional Court of South Africa, 2002(10) BCLR 1033.

11. *Soobramoney v. Minister of Health (Kwazulu-Natal)*, Constitutional Court of South Africa, 1997(12) BCLR 1696.

12. *South Africa v. Grootboom*, Constitutional Court of South Africa, 2000(11) BCLR 1169.

13. Tarantola, D., and Gruskin, S., Children Confronting HIV/AIDS: Charting the Confluence of Rights and Health, *Health and Human Rights* 1998; 3: 61–85; and Ngwena, C., The Recognition of Access to Health Care as a Human Right in South Africa: Is It Enough? *Health and Human Rights* 2000; 5: 27–44. *See also* Torres, M. A., The Human Right to Health, National Courts and Access to HIV/AIDS Treatment: A Case-Study from Venezuela, *Chicago Journal of International Law* 2002; 3: 105–115, and Yamin, A. E., Not Just a Tragedy: Access to Medications as a Right Under International Law, *Boston University International Law Journal* 2003; 21: 325–371

14. The right to health has been given more precise definition in a report of the Committee on Economic, Social, and Cultural Rights, the treaty entity formed

to help implement the International Covenant on Economic, Social, and Cultural Rights. The document is known as General Comment No. 14 and was issued in 2000. Among its most important provisions are the following:

1. Health is a fundamental human right indispensable for the exercise of other human rights . . .

4. . . . the right to health embraces a wide range of socio-economic factors that promote conditions in which people can lead a healthy life, and extends to the underlying determinants of health, such as food and nutrition, housing, access to safe and potable water and adequate sanitation, safe and healthy working conditions, and a healthy environment.

8. The right to health is not to be understood as a right to be *healthy*. The right to health contains both freedoms and entitlements. The freedoms include the right to control one's health and body, including sexual and reproductive freedom, and the right to be free from interference, such as the right to be free from torture, nonconsensual medical treatment and experimentation. By contrast, the entitlements include the right to a system of health protection which provides equality of opportunity for people to enjoy the highest attainable level of health.

11. . . . the right to health . . . [is] an inclusive right extending not only to timely and appropriate health care but also to the underlying determinants of health, such as access to safe and potable water and adequate sanitation, an adequate supply of safe food, nutrition and housing, healthy occupational and environmental conditions, and access to health-related education and information, including on sexual and reproductive health.

12. The right to health in all its forms and at all levels contains the following interrelated and essential elements, the precise application of which will depend on the condition prevailing in a particular State party:

   (a) *Availability*. Functioning public health and health-care facilities, goods and services, as well as programs, have to be available.

   (b) *Accessibility*. Health facilities, goods and services, have to be accessible to everyone without discrimination . . . physical accessibility . . . economic accessibility (affordability) . . . information accessibility . . .

   (c) *Acceptability* . . . All health facilities, goods and services must be respectful of medical ethics and culturally appropriate . . .

   (d) *Quality* . . . must also be scientifically and medically appropriate and of good quality. This requires, *inter alia*, skilled medical personnel, scientifically approved and unexpired drugs and hospital equipment, safe and potable water, and adequate sanitation.

17. The right to health facilities . . . [includes] the provision of . . . equal and timely access to basic preventive, curative, rehabilitative health

services and health education; regular screening programs; appropriate treatment of prevalent diseases, illnesses, injuries and disabilities, preferably at community level; the provision of essential drugs; and appropriate mental health treatment and care.

33. The right to health, like all human rights, imposes three types or levels of obligation on States parties: the obligations to *respect, protect, and fulfill* . . .

34. States are under the obligation to *respect* the right to health by, *inter alia*, refraining from denying or limiting equal access for all persons, including prisoners or detainees, minorities, asylum seekers and illegal immigrants, to preventive, curative and palliative health services; abstaining from enforcing discriminatory practices as a State policy; and abstaining from imposing discriminatory practices relating to women's health status and needs . . .

35. Obligations to *protect* include, *inter alia*, the duties of States to adopt legislation or to take other measures to ensuring equal access to health care and health-related services provided by third parties; to ensure that privatization of the health sector does not constitute a threat to the availability, accessibility, and quality of health facilities, goods and services; to control the marketing of medical equipment and medicines by third parties; and to ensure that medical practitioners and other health professionals meet appropriate standards of education, skill and ethical codes of conduct . . .

36. The obligation to *fulfill* requires States parties, *inter alia*, to give sufficient recognition to the right to health in the national political and legal systems, preferably by way of legislative implementation, and to adopt a national health policy with a detailed plan for realizing the right to health. States must ensure provision of health care, including immunization programs against the major infectious diseases, and ensure equal access for all to the underlying determinants of health, such as nutritiously safe food and potable drinking water, basic sanitation and adequate housing and living condition. Public health infrastructures should provide for sexual and reproductive health services, including safe motherhood, particularly in rural areas . . .

Core Obligations

43. . . . core obligations [minimum essential level of the right] include at least the following obligations:

   (a) To ensure the right of access to health facilities, goods and services on a nondiscriminatory basis, especially for vulnerable or marginalized groups;

   (b) To ensure access to the minimum essential food which is nutritionally adequate and safe, to ensure freedom from hunger to everyone;

(c) To ensure access to basic shelter, housing and sanitation, and an adequate supply of safe and potable water;

(d) To provide essential drugs, as from time to time defined under the WHO Action Program on Essential Drugs;

(e) To ensure equitable distribution of all health facilities, goods and services;

(f) To adopt and implement a national public health strategy and plan of action, on the basis of epidemiological evidence, addressing the health concerns of the whole population; the strategy and plan of action shall be devised, and periodically reviewed, on the basis of a participatory and transparent process; they shall include methods, such as right to health indicators and benchmarks, by which progress can be closely monitored; the process by which the strategy and plan of action are devised, as well as their content, shall give particular attention to all vulnerable or marginalized groups.

47. . . . a State party cannot, under any circumstances whatsoever, justify its noncompliance with the core obligations set out in paragraph 43, which are nonderogable.

15. DeCook, K. M., Mbori-Ngacha, D., and Marum, E., Shadow on the Continent: Public Health and HIV/AIDS in Africa in the 21st Century, *Lancet* 2002; 360: 67–72.

16. Benatar, S. R., Health Care Reform and the Crisis of HIV and AIDS in South Africa, *New England Journal of Medicine* 2004; 351: 81–91. After his 2002 trip to Africa with Bono to learn about the HIV/AIDS pandemic, Secretary of the Treasury Paul O'Neill returned to Washington convinced that clean water should be made a top priority in Africa, and that the U.S. government should commit at least to funding a demonstration well-drilling project in Ghana. His proposal was consistently and unceremoniously rejected, but O'Neill was correct to view clean water as a necessary condition for good health. Ron Suskind, *The Price of Loyalty: George W. Bush, the White House, and the Education of Paul O'Neill*, New York: Simon & Schuster, 2004, 253–269. President Mbeki continues to frustrate the Treatment Action Committee and others with his continued failure to put HIV/AIDS at the top of his administration's health agenda. Baleta, A., South African President Criticised for Lack of Focus on AIDS, *Lancet* 2004; 363: 541.

17. Mandela, N., Care Support and Destigmatization, Barcelona AIDS Conference, July 12, 2002.

18. Mukherjee, J., Basing Treatment on Rights Rather than Ability to Pay: 3 by 5, *Lancet* 2004; 363: 1071. This is a laudable and ambitious goal. But as Helen Gayle of the Gates Foundation has noted, even if WHO meets the goal, WHO will not be able to treat the five million new HIV infections that occur worldwide every year. Prevention efforts must be reinvigorated simultaneously with treatment. Altman, L., Report Urges More H.I.V. Prevention Along with Treatment, *New York Times*, June 11, 2004, A8.

Chapter 6

1. Immanuel Kant, *Perpetual Peace and Other Essays*, Indianapolis: Hackett Pub. Co. (Ted Humphrey, tr.), 1983, 86 (originally published in 1793). This chapter is adapted from Annas, G. J., Moral Progress, Mental Retardation, and the Death Penalty, *New England Journal of Medicine* 2002; 346: 1814–1818.

2. Annas, G. J., Killing with Kindness: Why the FDA Need Not Certify Drugs Used for Execution Safe and Effective, *American Journal of Public Health* 1985; 75: 1096–1099.

3. LeGraw, J. M., and Grodin, M. A., Health Professionals and Lethal Injection Execution in the United States, *Human Rights Quarterly* 2002; 24: 382–423; Troug, R. D., and Brennan, T. A., Participation of Physicians in Capital Punishment, *New England Journal of Medicine* 1993; 329: 1346–1350; and Curran, W. J., and Casscells, W., The Ethics of Medical Participation in Capital Punishment by Intravenous Drug Injection, *New England Journal of Medicine* 1980; 302: 226–230.

4. Melville, H., Billy Budd (in) *Great Short Works of Herman Melville,* New York: Harper & Row, 1966, 419.

5. Norman Mailer, *The Executioner's Song*, Boston: Little, Brown, 1979, 985–987.

6. *Wainwright v. Florida*, 477 U.S. 399 (1986).

7. *Atkins v. Virginia*, 536 U.S. 304 (2002).

8. *Rector v. Lockhart*, 727 F. Supp. 1285 (E.D. Ark. 1990); *Rector v. Clinton*, 398 Ark. 104, 823 S.W.2d 829 (1992).

9. Olgiati, C., The White House via Death Row, *The Guardian* (London), October 12, 1993, 18.

10. Frady, M., Death in Arkansas, *New Yorker*, February 22, 1993, 132.

11. *Penry v. Lynaugh*, 492 U.S. 302 (1989).

12. Root, J., Texas Gov. Bush Against Bill Banning Death Penalty for Retarded, *Ft. Worth Star-Telegram*, April 13, 1999, 12.

13. *Atkins v. Virginia*, 260 Va. 375, 534 S.E.2d 312 (2000).

14. *Weems v. U.S.*, 217 U.S. 349 (1910).

15. *Trop v. Dulles*, 356 U.S. 86 (1958).

16. *Penry*, supra note 11.

17. *Atkins*, supra note 7.

18. Jonathan Glover, *Humanity: A Moral History of The Twentieth Century*, New Haven, Conn.: Yale University Press, 2000.

19. Robert Drinan, *The Mobilization of Shame: A World View of Human Rights*, New Haven, Conn.: Yale University Press, 2001.

20. Shapiro, B., Rethinking the Death Penalty, *The Nation*, July 22–29, 2002, 14–19.

21. Kaminer, W., The Switch, *New York Times Magazine*, July 7, 2002, 7–8.

22. *See* Liptak, A., New Challenge for Courts: How to Define Retardation, *New York Times*, March 14, 2002, 20; and Jennings, D., Killer's Sentence Is Commuted: Perry's Action Is First Since Court Ruling on Retarded Inmates, *Dallas Morning News*, March 13, 2004, 3A.

23. British Medical Association, *The Medical Profession and Human Rights: Handbook for a Changing Agenda,* London: Zed Books, 2001, 163–191.

24. David F. Allen and Victoria S. Allen, *Ethical Issues in Mental Retardation: Tragic Choices/Living Hope,* Nashville: Abbingdon, 1979, 17–21.

25. Watt, M. J., and MacLean, W. E., Competency to Be Sentenced and Executed, *Ethics & Behavior* 2003; 13: 35, 39.

26. Turow, S., To Kill or Not to Kill, *New Yorker,* January 6, 2003, 40, 46.

27. LeGraw and Grodin, supra note 3.

Chapter 7

1. The facts of the Bijani case are drawn from contemporaneous news accounts.

2. Ben Carson interview with Renee Montagne, *NPR Morning Edition,* August 28, 2003. *See also* Grady, D., 2 Women, 2 Deaths and an Ethical Quandary, *New York Times,* July 15, 2003, D1, and Davis, J., Till Death Do Us Part, *Wired,* October 2003, 110–120.

3. Singapore Probe Clears Doctors of Criminal Liability on Iranian Twins' Death, AFX News Ltd., March 7, 2004, available at afx.com.

4. Thomasma, D. C., et al., The Ethics of Caring for Conjoined Twins: The Lakeberg Twins, *Hastings Center Report* 1996; 26(4): 4–12.

5. Rosato, J. L., Using Bioethics Discourse to Determine When Parents Should Make Health Care Decisions for Their Children: Is Deference Justified? *Temple Law Review* 2000; 73: 1–68.

6. Drake, D., The Twins Decision: One Must Die So One Can Live, *Philadelphia Inquirer,* October 16, 1977.

7. This section of the chapter is adapted from Annas, G. J., Conjoined Twins: The Limits of Law at the Limits of Life, *New England Journal of Medicine* 2001; 344: 1104–1108.

8. O'Neill, J. A., ed., Conjoined Twins (in) *Pediatric Surgery,* 5th ed., St. Louis: Mosby, 1998, 1925–1938.

9. Rosato, supra note 5.

10. *In re A* (children), 4 All E.R. 961 (C.A. 2000).

11. Cullen, K., In London, an Agonizing Decision, *Boston Globe,* September 11, 2000, A1, A8.

12. *Regina v. Dudley and Stephens,* [1884] 14 QBD 273.

13. A. W. Brian Simpson, *Cannibalism and the Common Law: The Story of the Tragic Last Voyage of the Mignonette and the Strange Legal Proceedings to Which It Gave Rise,* Chicago: University of Chicago Press, 1984.

14. Spitz, L., and Kiely, E., Success Rate for Surgery of Conjoined Twins, *Lancet* 2000; 356: 1765.

15. Laville, S., Mary Was Freed by Death, Says Father of Siamese Twins, *Daily Telegraph* (London), December 7, 2000, 1.

16. British Surgeon Reflects on Decision to Let Siamese Twin Die, *Toronto Star,* January 7, 2001, 1.

17. Bunyan, N., "Bright and Alert" Jodie Makes Rapid Progress, *Daily Telegraph* (London), December 16, 2000, 9.

18. Cramb, A., Village Children Mourn as Siamese Twin Is Laid to Rest, *Daily Telegraph* (London), January 20, 2001, 3.

19. Barton, F., Two Years On, A New Sister for Siamese Twin Gracie, Baby Rosie Named in Honor of Tiny Girl Who Had to Die, *Mail on Sunday*, August 25, 2002, 23.

20. William Styron, *Sophie's Choice*, New York: Vintage, 1992.

21. Annas, G. J., Siamese Twins: Killing One to Save the Other, *Hastings Center Report* 1987; 17(2): 27–29. Drake, supra note 6. Thomasma et al., supra note 4.

22. Bleich, J. D., Conjoined Twins, *Tradition* 1996; 31: 92–125.

23. Fuller, L., The Case of the Speluncean Explorers, *Harvard Law Review* 1949; 62: 616. *See also* The Case of the Speluncean Explorers: A Fiftieth Anniversary Symposium, *Harvard Law Review* 1999; 112: 1834.

24. Norwitz, E. R., et al., Separation of Conjoined Twins with the Twin Reversed: Arterial-Perfusion Sequencing after Prenatal Planning with Three-Dimensional Modeling, *New England Journal of Medicine* 2000; 343: 399–402.

25. *Re T*, 1 All E.R. 906 (1997) (liver transplant for a child may be refused because parents believe it is not in their child's interests, even though physicians disagree).

26. Courts have also adopted the principle of the double effect, an old religious doctrine, as legal doctrine. But how else could it be? If we did not have the doctrine of the double effect (or its functional equivalent), every time someone died on the operating table it would be homicide because the surgeon killed the patient. But we don't hold the patient's death against surgeons if their intent is to try to help the patient and they act in a medically reasonable and prudent manner, nor should we. If we believed that all that mattered was the outcome of the doctor's decision (and not intent or causation), stopping cardiopulmonary resuscitation (CPR) would be murder (or at least manslaughter) because the patient would die at the point when the physician stopped compressing the heart. But, of course, that is silly. We don't even think about homicide, let alone criminal charges, because we understand the goal of CPR is to try to revive the patient's spontaneous heartbeat and respiration. When that goal can't be met, it is only reasonable to stop, even though the patient dies. It does not mean the physician killed the patient.

Chapter 8

1. Leon Kass, *Life, Liberty and the Defense of Dignity: The Challenge for Bioethics*, San Francisco: Encounter Books, 2002, 57–65. Kass himself, in his role as head of the President's Council on Bioethics, has sought to redefine the field. In his words, "For the Council, 'bioethics' is not an ethics based on biology, but an ethics in the service of *bios*—of a life lived humanly, a course of life lived not merely physiologically, but also mentally, socially, culturally, politically, and spiritually." Kass, L. R., Being Human: An Introduction (in) The President's Council on Biothics, *Being Human: Readings from the President's Council on Bioethics*, Washington, D.C.: President's Council on Bioethics, 2003, xx–xxi. This

expansion is all to the good; and if the term "economically" was added to the description, could fit the human rights approach of the Universal Declaration of Human Rights as well (although this is almost certainly not what the Council or President Bush had in mind).

2. This chapter is adapted from Annas, G. J., A National Bill of Patient Rights, *New England Journal of Medicine* 1998; 338: 695–699.

3. *See* Annas, G. J., HIPAA Regulations: A New Era of Medical Record Privacy? *New England Journal of Medicine* 2003; 348: 1486–1490.

4. Paul Starr, *The Social Transformation of American Medicine*, New York: Basic Books, 1982, 388–393.

5. Informed consent and other patient rights are discussed in more detail in George J. Annas, *The Rights of Patients*, 3rd ed., Carbondale, Ill: Southern Illinois University Press, 2004.

6. *Roe v. Wade*, 410 U.S. 113 (1973).

7. Annas, G. J., Glantz, L. H., and Mariner, W. K., The Right of Privacy Protects the Doctor–Patient Relationship, *JAMA* 1990; 263: 858–861.

8. *See* supra note 5.

9. *See, e.g.,* Mark A. Rodwin, *Medicine, Money and Morals: Physicians' Conflicts of Interest*, New York: Oxford University Press, 1993.

10. Annas, G. J., Women and Children First, *New England Journal of Medicine* 1995; 333: 1647–1651.

11. Kertesz, L., HMO Makeover: Are Managed Care's Efforts to Overhaul Its Image Too Little, Too Late? *Modern Healthcare*, May 12, 1997, 36–46.

12. Kassirer, J. P., Managing Managed Care's Tarnished Image, *New England Journal of Medicine* 1997; 337: 338–339.

13. Pear, R., Three Big Health Plans Urge National Standards, *New York Times*, September 25, 1997, A1.

14. Pear, R., Panel of Experts Urges Broadening of Patient Rights, *New York Times*, October 23, 1997, A1; Advisory Commission on Consumer Protection and Quality in the Health Care Industry, *Consumer Bill of Rights and Responsibilities*, November 1997. Available at www.hcqualitycommission.gov/cborr.

15. Annas, G. J., Patients' Rights in Managed Care—Exit, Voice, and Choice, *New England Journal of Medicine* 1997; 337: 210–215.

16. Annas, G. J. and Healey, J., The Patient Rights Advocate: Redefining the Doctor–Patient Relationship in the Hospital Setting, *Vanderbilt Law Review* 1974; 27: 243–269, and supra note 5.

17. Furrow, B. R., Managed Care Organizations and Patient Injury: Rethinking Liability, *Georgia Law Review* 1997; 31: 419–509.

18. Mariner, W. K., Standards of Care and Standard Form Contracts: Distinguishing Patient Rights and Consumer Rights in Managed Care, *Journal of Contemporary Health Law & Policy* 1998; 15: 1–55.

Chapter 9

1. This chapter is adapted from Annas, G. J., The Last Resort: The Use of Physical Restraints in Medical Emergencies, *New England Journal of Medicine* 1999;

341: 1408–1412; and Annas, G. J., Testing Poor Pregnant Women for Cocaine: Physicians as Police Investigators, *New England Journal of Medicine* 2001; 344: 1729–1732.

2. The facts of this case are taken from the court opinion *Shine v. Vega*, 429 Mass. 456, 709 N.E.2d 58 (1999).

3. *Norwood Hospital v. Munoz*, 409 Mass 116, 564 N.E.2d 1017 (1991); *Matter of Conroy*, 98 N.J. 311, 486 A.2d 1209 (1985).

4. W. Page Keeton and William L. Prosser, *Torts*, 5th ed., St. Paul, Minn.: West Publishing Co., 1984, 117.

5. Annas, G. J., and Densberger, J. E., Competence to Refuse Medical Treatment: Autonomy vs. Paternalism, *Toledo Law Review* 1984; 15: 561–589.

6. Health Care Financing Administration, Department of Health and Human Services, Medicare and Medicaid Programs: Hospital Conditions of Participation, Patients' Rights, *Federal Register* 1998; 64: 36070–36089.

7. *Ibid. See also* Weiss, E. M., Hundreds of the Nations' Most Vulnerable Have Been Killed by the System Intended to Care for Them, *Hartford Courant*, October 11, 1998, A1.

8. *Truman v. Thomas*, 27 Cal. 3d 285, 165 Cal. Rptr. 505, 611 P.2d 902 (1980).

9. *Skinner v. Railway Labor Executives' Association*, 489 U.S. 602 (1989).

10. Siegel, B., In the Name of the Children, *Los Angeles Times Magazine*, August 7, 1994, 14.

11. Annas, G. J., Crack, Symbolism, and the Constitution, *Hastings Center Report* 1989; 19(3): 35–37.

12. *Ferguson v. City of Charleston*, 532 U.S. 67 (2001).

13. Supra note 10.

14. *Ferguson v. City of Charleston*, 186 F.3d. 469 (4th Cir. 1999).

15. *Veronia School Dist. 47J v. Acton*, 515 U.S. 646 (1995).

16. *Chandler v. Miller*, 520 U.S. 305 (1997).

17. *Ferguson v. City of Charleston*, 308 F.3d 380 (4th Cir. 2002).

18. Glantz, L. H., A Nation of Suspects: Drug Testing and the Fourth Amendment, *American Journal of Public Health* 1989; 79: 1427–1431.

19. Mariner, W. K., Glantz, L. H., and Annas, G. J., Pregnancy, Drugs, and the Perils of Prosecution, *Criminal Justice Ethics* 1990; 9: 30–41; Paltrow, L. M., When Becoming Pregnant Is a Crime, *Criminal Justice Ethics* 1990; 9: 41–47.

Physicians, of course, play many roles in society. Some, for example, are employed by governments to work in the prison system. In this role, physicians face the inherent problem of "dual loyalty" to their employer-the state and their patient-prisoner. In another decision by the U.S. Supreme Court, *U.S. v. Sell*, 539 U.S. 166 (2003), the Court ruled that under limited circumstances courts could authorize physicians to forcibly medicate prisoners who refused treatment (and were competent to refuse it), so that they might become competent to stand trial (which requires, among other things, the ability to cooperate with your lawyer and to understand the charges against you). The Court required judges to make four findings prior to authorizing forced medication: that important government interests were at stake, such as having a timely trial of a serious crime; that forced medication would significantly further the interest; that less intrusive alternatives are unlikely to achieve results; and that the administration of the drugs is "medically appropriate, i.e., in the patient's best medical interest in light of his medical condition."

As discussed in this chapter, it is never ethically acceptable to force treatment on a competent person—and the fact that a judge says that it is legal, does not change the medical ethics of the doctor–patient relationship. The good news in this otherwise distressing case is that the Court ruling does not force physicians to do anything inconsistent with medical ethics and their view of the patient's best medical interests. Of course, the Court cannot resolve the prison psychiatrist's dual loyalty conflict, and this decision only heightens it. Psychiatrists can lawfully (and ethically) respond by taking the Court at its word that accused prisoner should not be forcibly medicated unless the physician makes an independent assessment that medication is in the prisoner-patient's best medical interests. Thus the human rights way to read this opinion is to emphasize the Court's deferral to medical ethics. The legal realist, on the other hand, will assume that the state can hire psychiatrists who sincerely believe that it is almost always best for prisoners who are incompetent to stand trial to be medicated so that they can have their day in court (even though this is not a medical goal). In this way, both medical ethics and the needs of the state can seem to be satisfied. *See* Annas, G. J., Forcible Medication for Courtroom Competence: The Case of Charles Sell, *New England Journal of Medicine* 2004; 350: 2297–2301.

20. Frank, D. A., Augustyn, M., Knight, et al., Growth, Development, and Behavior in Early Childhood Following Prenatal Cocaine Exposure: A Systematic Review, *JAMA* 2001; 285: 1613–1625; Chavkin, W., Cocaine and Pregnancy—Time to Look at the Evidence, *JAMA* 2001; 285: 1626–1628.

21. *International Union v. Johnson Controls*, 499 U.S. 187 (1991).

22. Annas, G. J., Fetal Protection and Employment Discrimination—The *Johnson Controls* Case, *New England Journal of Medicine* 1991; 325: 740–743.

23. Valerie Green, *Doped Up, Knocked Up, and . . . Locked Up?: The Criminal Prosecution of Women Who Use Drugs During Pregnancy*, New York: Garland, 1993; Roberts, D., The Challenge of Substance Abuse for Family Preservation Policy, *Journal of Health Care Law & Policy* 1999; 3: 72–82.

Chapter 10

1. This chapter is adapted from Annas, G. J., Partial-Birth Abortion, Congress and the Constitution, *New England Journal of Medicine* 1998; 339: 279–283; and Annas, G. J., Partial Birth Abortion and the Supreme Court, *New England Journal of Medicine* 2001; 344: 152–156.

2. *Roe v. Wade*, 410 U.S. 113 (1973).

3. *Doe v. Bolton*, 410 U.S. 179 (1973).

4. *Planned Parenthood of Southeastern Pennsylvania v. Casey*, 502 U.S. 1056 (1992).

5. Remarks on returning without approval to the House of Representatives partial birth abortion legislation. *Weekly Compilation Presidential Documents* 32: 643–647, April 10, 1996.

6. Santorum, R., A Brief Life That Changed Our Lives Forever, *National Right to Life News*, May 23, 1997, 6–7.

7. Klein, J., The Senator's Dilemma, *New Yorker*, January 5, 1998, 30–35.

8. Vobejda, B., and Brown, D., Harsh Details Shift Tenor of Abortion Fight: Both Sides Bend Facts on Late-Term Procedure, *Washington Post*, September 17, 1996, A1.

9. American College of Obstetrics and Gynecology, *Statement on Intact Dilatation and Extraction*, January 12, 1997.

10. Gianelli, D., House Affirms AMA Stance on Abortion, *American Medical News*, July 7, 1997, 3.

11. Seelye, K. Q., Democratic Leader Proposes Measure to Limit Abortions, *New York Times*, May 9, 1997, A32.

12. Message to the House of Representatives Returning Without Approval Partial Birth Abortion Legislation, *Weekly Compilation Presidential Documents* 33: 1545, October 10, 1997.

13. *The Hope Clinic v. Ryan*, 195 F.3d 857 (7th Cir. 1999) (Posner, J. dissenting).

14. *Stenberg v. Carhart*, 530 U.S. 914 (2000).

15. *Carhart v. Stenberg*, 11 F. Supp. 2d 1099 (Neb. 1998)

16. *Stenberg v. Carhart*, 192 F.3d 1142 (1999)

17. *Lawrence v. Texas*, 539 U.S. 558 (2003)

18. Partial Birth Abortion Law of 2003 (S.3)

19. Stolberg, S. G., Senate Approves Bill to Prohibit Type of Abortion, *New York Times*, October 22, 2003, A1.

20. *Planned Parenthood v. Ashcroft*, 2004 U.S. Dist. LEXIS 9775 (June 1, 2004). *See also* Pear, R., and Lichtblau, E., Administration Sets Forth a Limited View on Privacy, *New York Times*, March 6, 2004, A8; Drazen, J. M., Inserting Government between Patient and Physician, *New England Journal of Medicine* 2004; 350: 178–179; and Greene, M. F., and Ecker, J. L., Abortion, Health, and the Law, *New England Journal of Medicine* 2004; 350: 184–186.

The administration's anti-woman behavior is even more intense on the international level, where the Bush administration has not only imposed a "gag rule" that permits its funding of women's health programs only to those who make no mention of abortion, but even attempted to have the language of the Cairo agreement under the Convention on the Elimination of All Forms of Discrimination Against Women (which the United States, along with 178 other countries, signed in 1994), amended to eliminate all references to "reproductive health" and "family planning services" at the Santiago meeting in 2004. As the *Boston Globe* described this action (taken on the same week as the president marked International Women's Day by claiming that the liberation of Afghanistan and Iraq "has given new rights and new hopes to women"): "For the Bush administration to claim that it cares for the human rights of women and then withdraw support for the Cairo agreement is a shocking abdication of responsibility and a

"selfish purposes such as enriching one's personal life, or the desire for heirs," and that having a child to be a donor should be accepted as long as we permit people to have children for worse motives. This not only makes the lowest common denominator of the reasons parents give for having their children an ethical norm, but also assumes that physicians should not take the interests of the potential children they are asked to help create into account when determining whether a medical procedure needed for their creation is ethically justified. It's another way of saying that physicians have ethical obligations only to their existing patients, not to the future children of their existing patients.

23. Developmental biologist Stuart Newman has noted that even if genetically-engineered human embryos could not produce viable children, these embryos could still be a valuable source of tissue for transplant if gestated for a time and then aborted. He has argued that we should take steps now to prevent this from happening (including, he believes, outlawing research cloning). Newman, S. A., Averting the Clone Age: Prospects and Perils of Human Developmental Manipulation, *Journal of Contemporary Health Law and Policy* 2003; 19: 431–463. In one of the few examples in which health law is actually out in front of scientific developments, current federal law already prohibits this practice by outlawing the designation of a recipient of fetal tissue by the donor. 42 U.S.C. sec. 280g-2(b) (prohibition regarding human fetal tissue). *See* Boyce, N., Parents Can Now Conceive Babies Whose Cells Can Cure a Sick Sibling. But What If the Pregnancy Goes Wrong? *U.S. News & World Report*, July 21, 2003, 48.

Concluding Remarks

1. George J. Annas and Michael Grodin, *The Nazi Doctors and the Nuremberg Code: Human Rights in Human Experimentation*, New York: Oxford University Press, 1992; and Shuster, E., Fifty Years Later: The Significance of the Nuremberg Code, *New England Journal of Medicine* 1997; 337: 1436–1440.

2. René Descartes, *The Philosophical Works of Descartes*, Cambridge: Cambridge University Press (E. S. Haldane and G. R. T. Ross, trs.), 1967, 211.

3. Jonathan Mann has also suggested the human rights tree model, with the UDHR as a trunk, although without including either bioethics or health law: "The Universal Declaration can be thought of as the trunk of the human rights tree, with the UN Charter as its roots. The two major branches, the two major International Covenants on Civil and Political Rights, and on Economic, Social and Cultural Rights, emerge from and expand upon the trunk with further elaboration through many important treaties and declarations." Mann, J., Human Rights and AIDS: The Future of the Pandemic, reprinted in Jonathan Mann et al., eds., *Health and Human Rights*, supra note 3, Chapter 5, 223.

4. *E.g.*, Albert Jonsen, *The Birth of Bioethics*, New York: Oxford University Press, 1992; David Rothman, *Strangers at the Bedside*, New York: Basic Books, 1991.

5. *See, e.g.*, Grodin, M., Annas, G. J., and Glantz, L. H., Medicine and Human Rights: A Proposal for International Action, *Hastings Center Report* 1993; 23(4): 8–12.

6. Beecher, H. K., Ethics and Clinical Research, *New England Journal of Medicine* 1966; 274: 1354–1360.

7. As Beecher put it in 1970: "The Nuremberg Code presents a rigid act of legalistic demands . . . The Declaration of Helsinki, on the other hand, presents a set of guides. It is an ethical as opposed to a legalistic document, and is thus a more broadly useful instrument than the one formulated at Nuremberg." Refshauge, W., The Place for International Standards in Conducting Research for Humans, *Bulletin of World Health Organization* 1977 (suppl.) 55: 133–135 (quoting Beecher).

8. Caplan, A. L., How Did Medicine Go So Wrong? (in) Arthur L. Caplan, ed., *When Medicine Went Mad: Bioethics and the Holocaust*, Totowa, N.J.: Humana Press, 1992, 53–92. An edited transcript of the Hastings Center conference, *Biomedical Ethics and the Shadow of Nazism*, was published as a supplement to the *Hastings Center Report* in August 1976. On the long relationship of national security and bioethics *see also* Moreno, J. D., Bioethics and the National Security State, *Journal of Law, Medicine & Ethics* 2004; 32: 1980–208.

9. A rewriting of the intellectual history of American bioethics is beyond the scope of this book, but my guess is that virtually anywhere one begins to dig in American bioethics, one will end with World War II. The best-known examples are from two of the field's intellectual founders: Jay Katz and Hans Jonas. Both were born in Germany and had family members killed in the Holocaust, and the bioethics-related writings of both grew out of their reflections on the war and the concentration camps. Jay Katz, for example, published what is still the leading text on human experimentation in 1972, and the Nuremberg Doctors' Trial was central to this collection of primary sources. His star student, and assistant in this project, Alex Capron, went on to be a leader in American bioethics himself, and I don't think it's an accident that he is currently the ethicist for one of the major "health and human rights" organizations in the world, the World Health Organization. Jay Katz himself was a member of two major U.S. bioethics panels that examined scandals: the Tuskegee Study Panel in 1972, and the President's Advisory Council of Human Radiation Experiments (1994–95). The Nuremberg Code was the centerpiece of the latter report—although attempts to distance bioethics from it continued. Hans Jonas was, of course, extremely prolific. His bioethics was also much broader than just medicine, and included the entire biosphere. Nonetheless, it was grounded in the Holocaust and the dehumanization of Auschwitz (where his mother was murdered). It is no accident that his own star pupil is now the head of America's bioethics council, Leon Kass.

10. The most comprehensive text on international human rights, and the one I rely on heavily in this conclusion, is Steiner and Alston, *International Human Rights in Context*, supra note 4, Chapter 2.

11. Fox, R., Medical Humanitarianism and Human Rights: Reflections on Doctors without Borders and Doctors of the World, reprinted in Jonathan Mann et al., eds., *Health and Human Rights: A Reader*, New York: Routledge, 1999, 417–435. With her colleague Judith Swazey, she has accused American bioethics of being based on "Anglo-American analytic philosophical thought [and thus projecting] an impoverished and skewed expression of our society's cultural tradition." Tom Beauchamp (coauthor with James Childress of the leading theoretical text on American bioethics, *Principles of Biomedical Ethics* (5th ed., New York: Oxford

University Press, 2001), recently described the Fox/Swazey thesis as "surprisingly influential," although given the isolation of American bioethics from the rest of the world, no surprise is warranted. Beauchamp, T. L., Does Ethical Theory Have a Future in Bioethics? *Journal of Law, Medicine & Ethics*, 2004; 32: 209–217. Fox and Swazey have had more uncomplimentary things to say about American bioethics. For example, "if bioethics is . . . more than medical—if it is an indicator of the general state of American ideas, values, and beliefs . . . then there is every reason to be worried about who we are, what we have become, what we know, and where we are going in a greatly changed and changing society and world." Fox, R. C., and Swazey, J. P., Medical Morality Is Not Bioethics: Medical Ethics in China and the United States, *Perspectives in Biology and Medicine* 1984; 27: 336–360. And on the narrow focus of American bioethics, "One of the most urgent value questions . . . [unexplored in bioethics] is whether as poverty, homelessness, and lack of access to health care increase in our affluent country, it is justifiable for American society to be devoting so much of its intellectual energy and human and financial resources to the replacement of human organs." Fox, R. C., and Swazey, J. P., Leaving the Field, *Hastings Center Report* 1992; 22(5): 9–15.

12. My colleague Michael Grodin and I followed up our conference on the 50th anniversary of the Nuremberg Code at the Holocaust Memorial Museum by founding our own physician NGO—but combining it with lawyers as well: Global Lawyers and Physicians. See http://www.glphr.org for details.

13. International Bioethics Committee, *Report of the IBC on the Possibility of Elaborating a Universal Instrument on Bioethics,* UNESCO, Paris, June 13, 2003, 1. My own view on the question of whether to draft a universal bioethics declaration is that the Universal Declaration of Human Rights already serves this purpose, and that we cannot do better. It is more constructive to put international efforts into instruments aimed at articulating standards for specific bioethics problem areas, such as genetics research. I agree, for example, with the spirit of the statement of former IBC chair, Ryuichi Ida of Japan, who noted of UNESCO's Universal Declaration on the Human Genome and Human Rights that it "has its place in the series of international instruments for the protection of human rights in the same way as the 1948 Universal Declaration of Human Rights, whose force is today universally recognized. The UNESCO declaration represents an extension of human rights protection to the field of biological sciences." Edmund Pellegrino has also strongly endorsed the centrality of the UDHR to medical ethics in the context of revelations about how physicians were used for torture under the Iraq dictatorship:

> National and international medical associations must examine more closely the implications of becoming instruments of anything other than the healing purposes for which the profession is ordained . . . This issue . . . must become a global issue if the United Nations' Universal Declaration of Human Rights is to maintain significance. With such powerful tools [advances in biotechnology that could be used for torture] in hand, will the medical profession remain a moral enterprise even in the face of threatening emergencies?

Pellegrino, E. D., Medical Ethics Suborned by Tyranny and War, *JAMA* 2004; 291: 1505–1506.

14. For an excellent account of the origins of the Declaration, *see* Mary Ann Glendon, *A World Made New: Eleanor Roosevelt and the Universal Declaration of Human Rights*, New York: Random House, 2001.

15. President's Council on Bioethics, *Beyond Therapy: Biotechnology and the Pursuit of Happiness*, Washington, D.C.: President's Council on Bioethics, 2004. *See also* Robert Pollack, *The Missing Moment*, New York: Houghton Mifflin Co., 1999, 155–160.

16. *See, e.g.*, Harold Hongju Koh, Introduction of U.S. Department of State (in) *1999 Country Reports on Human Rights Practices*, Washington, D.C.: U.S. Dept. of State, 2000 ("in the new millennium, there are at least three universal 'languages': money, the Internet, and democracy and human rights"). *See also* Knowles, L. P., The Lingua Franca of Human Rights and the Rise of a Global Bioethic, *Cambridge Quarterly of Healthcare Ethics* 2001; 10: 253–263; and Thomasma, D. C., Proposing a New Agenda: Bioethics and International Human Rights, *Cambridge Quarterly of Healthcare Ethics* 2001; 10: 299–310; and Andorno, R., Biomedicine and International Human Rights Law: In Search of a Global Consensus, *Bulletin of World Health Organization* 2002; 80(12): 959–963. *And see* supra note 1, Chapter 8.

An international human rights approach is also consistent with Kant's views on enlightenment in the context of the entire human species, all of whose members "have an interest in the preservation of the whole" giving rise to the hope that "after many revolutions of reform, nature's supreme objective—a universal *cosmopolitan state*, the womb in which all of the human species' original capacities will be developed—will at last come to be realized" (emphasis in original). Immanuel Kant, *Perpetual Peace and Other Essays*, Indianapolis: Hackett Pub. Co. (Ted Humphrey, tr.), 1983, 38 (originally published in 1784). Kant's philosophy supports the concept of universal human rights, and of giving all human beings the status of "world citizens." Giovanna Borradori, *Philosophy in a Time of Terror: Dialogues with Jurgen Habermas and Jacques Derrida*, Chicago: University of Chicago Press, 2003, 55.

The father of American pragmatism, philosopher John Dewey (the favorite philosopher of the first chair of a national bioethics commission in the United States, physician Kenneth Ryan, among others) espoused a frontier pragmatism that is also perfectly at home with the concept of equal humans freely moving toward a better world by virtue of their intelligence and experience. "It is [American pragmatism's] faith in the power of free intelligence to work its way, item by item and day by day, to that union . . . which the United Nations purports and the Universal Declaration of Human Rights affirms." Kallen, H. M., John Dewey and the Spirit of Pragmatism (in) Sidney Hook, ed., *John Dewey: Philosopher of Science and Freedom: A Symposium*, New York: Dial Press, 1950, 45.

17. Salman Rushdie, *Step Across This Line: Collected Nonfiction 1992–2002*, New York: Random House, 2002, 381.

18. Saramago, J., From Justice to Democracy by Way of the Bells, closing speech given at the World Social Forum, Porto Alegré, Brazil, January 22, 2002, available at http://www.terraincognita.50megs.com/saramagoalt.html. *See also* Farmer, P. and Campos, N. G., New Malaise: Bioethics and Human Rights in the Global Era, *Journal of Law, Medicine & Ethics* 2004; 32: 243–251.

Index